Pediatric Rheumatology
in Clinical Practice

Ronald M. Laxer • David D. Sherry
Philip J. Hashkes

Pediatric Rheumatology
in Clinical Practice

Second Edition

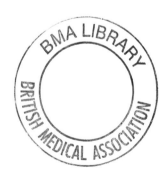

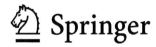 Springer

Ronald M. Laxer
Hospital for Sick Children
University of Toronto
Toronto, Ontario
Canada

Philip J. Hashkes
Pediatric Rheumatology Unit
Shaare Zedek Medical Center
Jerusalem
Israel

David D. Sherry
Children's Hospital of
Philadelphia
Philadelphia, PA
USA

ISBN 978-3-319-13098-9   ISBN 978-3-319-13099-6   (eBook)
DOI 10.1007/978-3-319-13099-6

Library of Congress Control Number: 2016941878

Printed on acid-free paper

This Springer imprint is published by Springer Nature
The registered company is Springer-Verlag London Ltd.

Preface

Pediatric rheumatology is a relatively new specialty, with many fascinating conditions peculiar to young people, virtually all of which are considered "orphan" diseases that are only rarely encountered by the generalist and therefore often present as diagnostic and therapeutic dilemmas. The popularity of the initial edition of this handbook suggested the need for a resource to fill the knowledge gap by assisting the pediatrician, the general practitioner, as well as rheumatologists with an interest in pediatric rheumatology, in the diagnosis and management of these diseases and problems. The emphasis has been placed on clinical presentation and how to arrive at a diagnosis, and an up-to-date management plan, using tables, algorithms, and figures as visual aids. Brief background information on the etiology is also provided. In this second edition we have added new knowledge accumulated since the first edition was published in 2007, particularly on new treatments for juvenile idiopathic arthritis and advances in the field of autoinflammatory diseases. We have also added a new chapter on tumors involving the musculoskeletal system. We sincerely hope that the information herein will help decrease the impact of these conditions on the children and their families by timely diagnosis and early intervention.

Toronto, ON, Canada   Ronald M. Laxer
Philadelphia, PA, USA   David D. Sherry
Jerusalem, Israel   Philip J. Hashkes

Contents

Chapter 1
General Presentation of Musculoskeletal Problems in Childhood

1.1 Introduction

The rheumatic diseases in children range from affecting a very isolated part of the body to including almost every organ and body system. The key to making a diagnosis usually rests in the patient's history and physical examination. Paramount is the knowledge of what normal is, especially in the musculoskeletal examination. Laboratory and imaging studies help substantiate a diagnosis, and at times are essential, so determining the most efficacious use of these resources is vital. However, there exist children who defy our classification systems and will have features of several concurrent rheumatic diseases (overlap syndromes) or just one part of a disease. It may take years before enough manifestations of their disease develop to allow a diagnosis to be definitively made (if ever). Additionally, some children will evolve from one diagnostic category into another so one needs to always be vigilant when caring for children with rheumatic illnesses.

1.2 Rheumatologic History

A typical rheumatologic history is shown in Table 1.1. Determining if a condition is inflammatory is generally the first step. Inflammation is characterised by pain, warmth, redness, swelling, and limitation of function. Some inflammatory

R.M. Laxer et al., *Pediatric Rheumatology in Clinical Practice*, 1
DOI 10.1007/978-3-319-13099-6_1,
© Springer-Verlag London 2016

TABLE 1.1 Rheumatologic history

Present illness

Chief complaint? (could be pain, fever, rash, fatigue, dry mouth, or other rheumatic symptoms)

Present medications and treatments?

Recent past medications and treatments? (for this condition and for other conditions)

Location of pain?

Details of onset: acute, gradual, traumatic?

Duration of pain?

Severity of pain: getting better or worse?

Quality of pain: stabbing, burning, freezing, aching, spasms, crushing?

Particular time of day that it is worse or better?

Specifically, morning, evening, or nocturnal pain?

Does it radiate, migrate, or is it episodic?

It is hot or cold to the touch?

Does it look different or swollen?

Does it interfere with functioning? School attendance, chores, recreation, activities of daily living (dressing, eating, bathing, toileting)?

Does anything make it better or worse? Medications, rubbing, ice, heat, activity, rest, distraction?

Between 0 and 10, how much does it hurt? (or other pain scale such as Faces Scale). Right now, highest and lowest in the past week?

Associated symptoms? Fever, rash, weight change, weakness, sleep disturbance, depression, anxiety, behavior change, cough, vision or hearing changes, headache, abdominal pain, diarrhea, dizziness, unable to concentrate?

(continued)

TABLE 1.1 (continued)

Past history

   Allergies

   Similar problem in the past?

   Immunization history, especially measles and hepatitis B

   Hospitalisations and surgeries

   Recent eye examination?

Social history

   Any new life events? Divorce, moving, school changes, family member changes?

   Any change in grade in school and school performance?

   Living with whom?

   Travel outside the area? Where? Tick bite? Diarrhea?

Family history

   Family members with rheumatic disease (SLE, arthritis, IBD, reactive arthritis, ankylosing spondylitis), psoriasis, back pain or spasms, even if family members know why they have back pain, heel spurs or heel pain, iritis, fibromyalgia, tuberculosis

   Family friends with chronic pain or infections such as tuberculosis. Family member with early stroke or heart attack, deep vein thrombosis or miscarriage?

Review of systems

   Complete review needs to be taken, but specific to the rheumatic diseases include dry mouth or eyes, hair coming out, trouble swallowing, hoarse voice, frequent infections, genital sores or discharge, fingers turning colors in the cold, easy bruising, hearing changes, conjunctivitis, eye pain, vision changes, rashes, photosensitivity, allodynia, and weight loss

conditions only have one or two of these findings, and 25 % of children with oligoarthritis report no pain. Morning stiffness and gelling (stiffness after being still such as in a car ride) are important indicators of inflammation. However, pain and loss of function are frequent in those without inflammation so the entire picture needs to be considered before arriving at a conclusion.

1.3   Family History

Many of the rheumatic diseases have a genetic basis so family history takes on an increased importance, including ethnic extraction, since many conditions are more frequent in select groups. One of the more common subtle clues is lower back pain that goes unreported because it is presumed to be due to trauma. Many parents with spondyloarthropathy have been diagnosed because the child presents with enthesitis-related arthritis.

1.4   Social History

Social history is important especially in children with amplified musculoskeletal pain and those with chronic conditions, which will impact on the family and social functioning of the child. There is an emotional impact of all illnesses on the entire family, especially those that are chronic, life threatening, or disabling.

1.5   Past History

Past history may reveal that the problem at hand is a recurrent problem, or is a consequence of a prior event or travel to an area endemic for particular infections.

1.6   General Physical Examination

The rheumatic diseases can affect a person wherever there is a blood vessel or where there isn't, so a complete examination is mandatory. Special rheumatic investigations include a careful examination of the skin (including nails, nailfold capillaries, hair), eyes (cornea, iritis, retina), ears (hearing), all mucous membranes, teeth (apical caries), lymph nodes (epitrochlear, axillary, and supraclavicular if malignancy is suspected), vessels (pulses and bruits), testes, heart (murmurs and rubs), lungs (dullness, rubs), abdomen (tenderness, peritonism, ascites, enlarged organs), nervous system (muscle tone, bulk, strength, reflexes, cranial nerves, mental states, cerebral function, sensation), and, of course, the joints, tendons, bursae and entheses. This is in addition to observing the child and family emotional interactions that may influence the child's care and diagnosis.

1.7 Joint Examination

The joint examination is probably the hardest part to master and even seasoned rheumatologists will differ in their assessment of which joints are inflamed. Careful attention should be given to each joint and each joint should be examined for swelling and warmth. Rapid joint movement will elicit guarding, an early sign of inflammation. Special mention should be made about several finer points of the joint examination. The temporomandibular joint (TMJ) can be destroyed painlessly, so close attention should be given to the jaw excursion and any deviation investigated (Fig. 1.1a–d). The tooth-to-tooth gap should be at least the width of the child's index, middle, and ring fingers held together (Fig. 1.2). Have the child look up in order to observe for asymmetrical jaw growth. The first range to be limited in cervical spine disease is extension (check by having the child squeeze your finger between the base of their neck and occiput). Elbows are best felt by holding the arm from the medial side and palpating just lateral to the olecranon as you extend the elbow (Fig. 1.3). Lower back range of motion is ascertained by the modified Schober test. This is done by making a mark on the spine at the superior border of the dimples of Venus (posterior superior iliac spine) and marks 10 cm cephaled and 5 cm caudad to this mark while the patient is standing (Fig. 1.4). The resulting 15 cm segment is measured when the patient leans forward and should expand to 21 cm or more. The entheses, where tendons attach to bone, need to be palpated directly, especially those shown in Fig. 1.5.

1.8   Laboratory and Imaging Studies

Laboratory and imaging studies will be discussed with each clinic entity, but there are some general rules. Only order tests where you think the results may assist with the diagnosis. This is especially true regarding an antinuclear antibody (ANA) test in a child without arthritis or in whom you do not suspect lupus; up to 15 % of normal children have a positive ANA

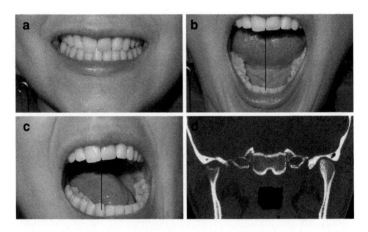

FIGURE 1.1 Normal and abnormal temporomandibular joint excursion (or jaw gait): the gap between the upper two central incisors should be compared to the lower teeth with the mouth closed (**a**) and remain in the relative same horizontal plane with the mouth open (**b**). Note that in (**c**) the jaw deviates to the child's right. Computerized tomography shows destruction of the right temporomandibular joint (**d**)

test [1]. Subsequent evaluation leads to unnecessary cost and angst. Another example is a very high alkaline phosphatase due to benign transient hyperphosphatasemia, which is common in young normal children, but also occurs in older children and even adults. A repeat test is usually required to support a diagnosis. Most criteria require repeated abnormalities separated by minimal periods of time such as rheumatoid factor (RF) in juvenile idiopathic arthritis (JIA) and low blood counts in systemic lupus erythematosus (SLE). The most important tests should be confirmed over time. Tests can be altered by treatment such as an increased erythrocyte sedimentation rate (ESR) after administration of intravenous immunoglobulin (IVIG). Imaging is never as good as histology and all imaging techniques can be false or misinterpreted.

The patterns of illness can be divided into systemic and localized, and each of these can be chronic or acute (Table 1.2). Usually it is not too difficult to tell the difference, but within

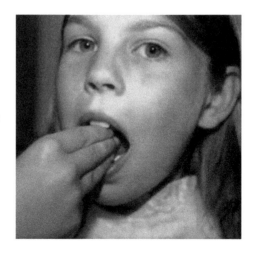

FIGURE 1.2 A quick way to check for adequate temporomandibular joint excursion: The patient should be able to get his or her own three fingers into the mouth

FIGURE 1.3 Proper
position of the
hand to examine
the elbow: An
effusion would be
felt under the mid-
dle finger of the
examiner's hand
when the elbow is
extended

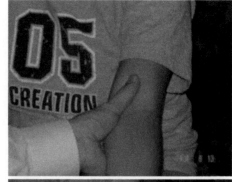

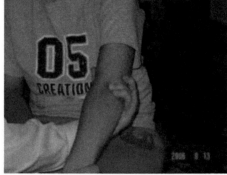

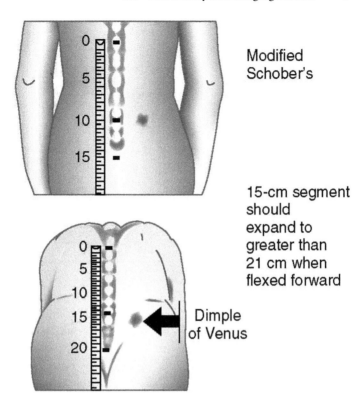

FIGURE 1.4 Modified Schober test: a mark 10 above and 5 cm below the superior border of the dimples of Venus should expand to 21 cm or more

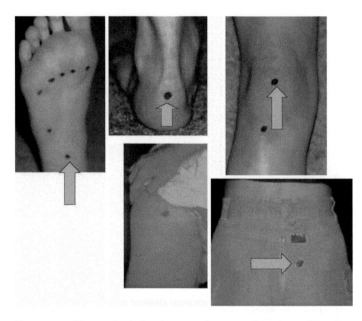

FIGURE 1.5 The enthesis is where tendons attach to bone. The sites that are the most commonly involved entheses in enthesitis-related arthritis are shown with *arrows*

each of these broad areas there are subtle differences between the illnesses.

1.9   Clues to the Diagnosis

There are often important clues to the diagnosis (Table 1.3). For example, JIA is almost never associated with a red joint. Keeping these points in mind will help one more quickly establish a differential diagnosis and help one select laboratory and imaging studies in a thoughtful and effective manner. Since there are many variations on the theme one cannot be locked into a "cookbook" approach to diagnosis or treatment and each child needs individual tailoring of diagnostic tests and therapy.

TABLE 1.2 Patterns of illness

Systemic		Localized	
Acute	**Chronic**	**Acute**	**Chronic**
Polyarthritis	Polyarthritis	Reactive arthritis	Oligoarthritis
Acute rheumatic fever	RF+ polyarthritis JIA	Hemarthrosis	Osteoid osteoma
Kawasaki	Takayasu	Toxic synovitis	Polyarthritis
Dermatomyositis	Dermatomyositis	Lyme	Lyme
Systemic JIA	Systemic JIA	SCFE	SCFE
Septic arthritis	Diffuse pain syndromes	Localised pain syndromes	Localized pain syndromes
Malignancy	Scleroderma	Legg–Calvé–Perthes	Legg–Calvé–Perthes
SLE	SLE	Enthesitis-related arthritis	Enthesitis-related arthritis
MCTD	MCTD	Psoriatic JIA	Psoriatic JIA
Granulomatosis with polyangiitis (Wegener)	Granulomatosis with polyangiitis (Wegener)	Iridocyclitis	Iridocyclitis

(continued)

TABLE 1.2 (continued)

Systemic		Localized	
Acute	Chronic	Acute	Chronic
Polyangiitis	Polyangiitis	Osgood–Schlatter	Osgood–Schlatter
Autoinflammatory syndromes	Autoinflammatory syndromes	PVNS	PVNS
IgA vasculitis (Henoch-Schönlein purpura)			Linear morphea
			Idiopathic chondrolysis
			Erythromelalgia
			Metabolic storage diseases

JIA juvenile idiopathic arthritis, *SLE* systemic lupus erythematosus, *PVNS* pigmented villonodular synovitis, *SCFE* slipped capital femoral epiphysis

Table 1.3   Clues to help construct a differential diagnosis

Clues	Diagnoses to consider			
Sick	Septic arthritis	Kawasaki	Inflammatory bowel disease	
	Osteomyelitis	Reactive arthritis	SLE/MCTD/JDM	
	Acute rheumatic fever		Sarcoidosis	Leukemia
	Neuroblastoma	Serum sickness	Lyme	
	Primary vasculitis	Pyomyositis	Autoinflammatory syndromes	
	Hypertrophic pulmonary osteoarthropathy		Systemic JIA	
Red joint	Septic arthritis	Osteomyelitis	Leukemia	
	Acute rheumatic fever	Reactive arthritis	Kawasaki	
	SLE/MCTD			

(continued)

TABLE 1.3 (continued)

Clues	Diagnoses to consider		
Hip pain	Septic arthritis	Idiopathic chondrolysis	Osteoid osteoma
	Spondyloarthropathy	Legg–Calvé–Perthes	Slipped capital femoral epiphysis
	Toxic synovitis	Leukemia	Oligoarthritis
Pain behind the knee	Benign hypermobility syndrome	Synovial cyst	Growing pains
Enthesitis	Spondyloarthropathy: ankylosing spondylitis, reactive arthritis, inflammatory bowel disease, psoriasis, enthesopathy without arthritis	Enthesitis-related arthritis	

Enthesalgia	Aseptic necrosis: Köhler–tarsal navicular; Kienböck–carpel lunate; Frieberg–second or third metatarsal head	Avulsion fracture: Osgood–Schlatter–tibal tuberosity; Sinding–Larsen–Johansson–patella	
Dactylitis	Psoriatic arthritis	Sickle cell anemia	Enthesitis-related arthritis
Rash	Acute rheumatic fever	Serum sickness	SLE/MCTD
	Dermatomyositis	Psoriasis	Inflammatory bowel disease
	Kawasaki	Reactive arthritis	IgA vasculitis (Henoch-Schönlein purpura)
	Primary vasculitis	Lyme	Gonorrhea
	Meningococcus	Viral	Rocky Mountain spotted fever
	Autoinflammatory syndromes	Systemic JIA	

(continued)

TABLE 1.3 (continued)

Clues	Diagnoses to consider		
Not walking	*see under* Sick and monarticular pain/arthritis, plus fracture[a]	Osteoid osteoma	Amplified musculoskeletal pain
	Discitis	Spinal cord tumor	Myositis
	Systemic JIA	Polyarthritis	
Neurologic symptoms	Cerebral palsy	Lyme	SLE/MCTD
	Polyarteritis nodosa	Kawasaki	Sarcoidosis
	Systemic infection	Systemic JIA	Cerebral vasculitis
Clubbing	Cystic fibrosis	Familial	Inflammatory bowel disease
	Hypertrophic pulmonary osteoarthropathy		

Monarticular pain/arthritis	Septic arthritis	Hemophilia	Pigmented villonodular synovitis
	Trauma[a]	Thorn (foreign body)	Aseptic necrosis
	Osteoid osteoma	Reactive	Osteochondritis dissecans
	Osteoid sarcoma	Viral	Leukemia (especially hip)
	Oligoarthritis		
Bone pain	Leukemia	Fracture[a]	Sickle cell anemia
	Osteoid osteoma (night pain)		
Migratory arthritis	Acute rheumatic fever	Lyme	Viral
	Palindromic rheumatism	Leukemia	

(continued)

TABLE 1.3 (continued)

Clues	Diagnoses to consider		
Episodic arthritis	Thalassemia	Sickle cell	Familial Mediterranean fever
	Palindromic rheumatism	Hyperlipidemia	Crystal disease
	Leukemia		
Raynaud phenomenon	Scleroderma	SLE	MCTD
	Primary, unassociated with other diseases (can be familial)		
Allodynia	Amplified musculoskeletal pain	Shingles	Infection
	Apprehension		
Incongruent affect	Amplified musculoskeletal pain		

Cyanosis/cold	Amplified musculoskeletal pain	Raynaud phenomenon
	Arterial occlusion (APLS, SLE, MCTD, scleroderma, vasculitis)	

[a]One must consider the possibility of nonaccidental injury with fractures and trauma in children

SLE systemic lupus erythematosus, *MCTD* mixed connective tissue disease, *JIA* juvenile idiopathic arthritis, *JDM* juvenile dermatomyositis, *APLS* antiphospholipid antibody syndrome

1.10   Etiology

Regarding etiology, the causes of the rheumatic diseases are unknown unless you include septic arthritis and osteomyelitis, Lyme disease or those with specific genetic defects. We know the triggers for acute rheumatic fever and some for reactive arthritis, and the genes involved in most of the recurrent fever syndromes described thus far.

1.11   Prevalence

The prevalence of the rheumatic illness varies between racial groups and geography and there are scant data regarding the rarer conditions [2–4]. Table 1.4 summarizes the numbers of children with various rheumatic illnesses given a population of one million children.

TABLE 1.4 Number of children with different rheumatic diseases expected in a population of 1 million children

Illness	Expected number	Sex predilection	Racial predilection
Juvenile idiopathic arthritis total	2050	Overall F > M	White > Asian > Black
Oligoarthritis	600	4F:1M	White
Polyarthritis RF+	100	4+F:1M	White
Polyarthritis RF−	400	3F:1M	White
Systemic	100	F = M	All
Psoriatic arthritis	150	F slightly > M	90 % White
Enthesitis-related	500	F < M	White, Native American, Asian

(continued)

TABLE 1.4 (continued)

Illness	Expected number	Sex predilection	Racial predilection
Other	200	Probably F > M	White
Systemic lupus erythematosus	150	5–10F: 1M	Black, Asian, Hispanic
Juvenile dermatomyositis/ polymyositis	15	3F: 1M	White
Scleroderma	15	2F: 1M systemic, F = M localized	All equal
Vasculitis syndromes	100–200	Depends on diagnosis	Variable depending on diagnosis
Lyme disease	Highly variable	F = M	Limited geographically to the tick vector, rural > urban
Autoinflammatory (recurrent fever) syndromes	Variable on racial population	Depends on diagnosis	Depends on diagnosis
Acute rheumatic fever	5	F – M	Much higher in developing countries
Pain syndromes	200–400	4F: 1M	Maybe higher in upper socioeconomic groups

For many of these conditions, the numbers are estimated based on the populations of pediatric rheumatology clinics, not on formal population studies [1–3]

References

1. Malleson PN, Mackinnon MJ, Sailer-Hoeck M, Spencer CH. Review for the generalist: the antinuclear antibody test in children – when to use it and what to do with a positive titer. Pediatr Rheumatol Online J. 2010;8:27.
2. Bowyer S, Roettcher P. Pediatric rheumatology clinic populations in the United States: results of a 3 year survey. Pediatric Rheumatology Database Research Group. J Rheumatol. 1996;23:1968–74.
3. Malleson PN, Fung MY, Rosenberg AM. The incidence of pediatric rheumatic diseases: results from the Canadian Pediatric Rheumatology Association Disease Registry. J Rheumatol. 1996;23:1981–7.
4. Symmons DP, Jones M, Osborne J, Sills J, Southwood TR, Woo P. Pediatric rheumatology in the United Kingdom: data from the British Pediatric Rheumatology Group National Diagnostic Register. J Rheumatol. 1996;23:1975–80.

Chapter 2
General Principles of Management

2.1 Introduction

The aim of any therapy is to address the cause and/or mechanisms of the disease. This may be done using drugs and structured rehabilitation. In some cases, psychotherapy is required. It is important to recognize that disease pathology can cause alteration in behavior, especially in the very young who are unable to articulate symptoms. Chronic illness can disturb the family dynamic and the child's education and development. Therefore, an age appropriate multidisciplinary approach is frequently required to restore function and fully integrate the child back into his/her family, school and peer group. Transition to adolescence and adulthood needs to be structured and started in early adolescence [1]. Ideally, all therapeutic methods should be evidence based. However, inherent in all therapy is an element of trial and error, as there are always individual variations due to each person's unique genetic and metabolic background. Currently, physicians arrive at their preferred option often through a Bayesian approach, maximizing the probability of success from published data, as well as from past and collective experiences. However in the future personal treatment plans will be established based on the precision medicine initiative centered on studying individual characteristics, for example, genetic polymorphisms, epigenetics and the microbiome. Initial research

R.M. Laxer et al., *Pediatric Rheumatology in Clinical Practice*, 23
DOI 10.1007/978-3-319-13099-6_2,
© Springer-Verlag London 2016

into precision medicine has been published in pediatric rheumatology [2], and it is expected that this will rapidly increase.

2.2   Inflammatory/Autoimmune Diseases

This group comprises the juvenile idiopathic arthritides (JIA), the multisystem inflammatory diseases, such as systemic lupus erythematosus (SLE), juvenile dermatomyositis (JDM), scleroderma, vasculitis and the autoinflammatory (recurrent fever) syndromes, many of which have a genetic mutation identified affecting the homeostasis of the inflammatory, mainly innate immunity, network. Individual descriptions of these diseases and their treatment algorithms are described in more detail in this book. Clinical recommendations/guidelines for some have been published, e.g., treatment of JIA by the American College of Rheumatology (ACR) and other national organizations, for lupus nephritis by the European League Against Rheumatism (EULAR) [3–5]. Anti-inflammatory drugs that suppress the action or synthesis of mediators of inflammation, are the first options for treating these diseases. The mode of action of many synthetic medications is not entirely clear and in vitro experiments have shown cellular effects as well as suppression of proinflammatory cytokines. Non-steroidal anti-inflammatory drugs (NSAIDs) that inhibit cyclooxygenase 1 and 2, traditionally considered first-line therapy, are presently used more as symptomatic rather than as disease modifying treatment. Corticosteroids are used systemically in many rheumatic diseases, especially at onset and during flares. In arthritis intra-articular corticosteroid injections are employed much more frequently than systemic use. In order to minimize chronic use of corticosteroids other synthetic disease modifying anti-rheumatic drugs (DMARDs), immunosuppressive and biologic medications are used, often very early in the disease course. DMARDs include methotrexate, sulfasalazine, leflunomide and hydroxychloroquine. Immunosuppressive medications such as azathioprine, mycophenolate mofetil, cyclophosphamide and cyclosporine A are used primarily in SLE, vasculitis and severe dermatomyositis. An increasing number of anti-cytokine biologic agents, including tumor necrosis factor (TNF), interleukin (IL)-1 and IL-6 inhibitors have been approved for use in pediatric rheumatology. Other anti-cytokine agents, including IL-17 and IL-23 inhibitors have been studied in adult rheumatic diseases. Other biologic medications are based on depleting certain populations of lymphocytes thought to be pathogenic (anti CD-20 mature B-cells/rituximab), or inhibiting T-cell functions (abatacept). Intracellular inflammatory signaling pathway inhibitors such as those that oppose Janus kinase (JAK) and signal transducer and activator of transcription (STAT) are being studied in children. Intravenous immunoglobulins are used primarily in Kawasaki disease and dermatomyositis. Other unclassified medications include thalidomide used in severe mucocutaneous Behçet disease and SLE and colchicine for familial Mediterranean fever and selected other autoinflammatory syndromes (see Tables 2.1 and 2.2). Autologous stem cell transplantation has been used in severe systemic JIA, SLE and systemic sclerosis, with some success, but this is a treatment with considerable morbidity and a mortality rate of around 5–10 % in the case of JIA and should still be regarded as experimental. Specific treatment for individual diseases will be covered within the individual chapters.

2.3   Pain in Inflammatory Diseases

The pain threshold is lowered in children with JIA and, clinically, one often encounters secondary pain amplification in these children [6]. Relative lack of physical activity, sleep disturbances related to pain and medications and the release of prostanoids and the proinflammatory cytokine IL-1 has been shown to cause pain and lower pain threshold. These mediators have direct effects on the central nervous system, in addition to their inflammatory actions peripherally. There

TABLE 2.1 Major anti-inflammatory/immunomodulatory drugs currently used in pediatric rheumatology targeting soluble mediators

Drug type	Mode of action
NSAID	Cyclooxygenase 1 and 2 inhibition
Corticosteroids	Suppress inflammatory cytokine production
Methotrexate	Suppress inflammatory cytokine production, increase local adenosine release and accumulation thus inhibiting neutrophil adhesion, inhibits dihydrofolate reductase, inhibits lymphocyte proliferation in high doses
Thalidomide	Inhibits cytokine secretion (especially TNF)
TNF inhibitors[a]	Blocks the action of TNF (inflammation, downstream cytokines, T and B cell signaling, and T cell proliferation)
IL-1 inhibitors[b]	Blocks the activity of IL-1 (inflammation, fever, downstream cytokines)
Anti-sIL-6R	Tocilizumab: a humanized monoclonal antibody that blocks cell signaling by the complex of IL-6/IL-6R (downstream cytokines, hepcidin, osteoclasts, growth inhibition)

NSAID non-steroidal anti-inflammatory drugs, *TNF* tumor necrosis factor, *IL-1* interleukin 1, *IL-6* interleukin 6, *IL-6R* interleukin 6 receptor, *sIL-6R* soluble IL-6R

[a]Infliximab, adalimumab, golimumab and certolizumab pegol are recombinant chimeric (infliximab) or humanized antibodies to TNFα; etanercept is a recombinant form of the naturally occurring sTNF receptor and traps/blocks TNFα

[b]Anakinra is an IL-1 receptor antagonist; rilonacept is a recombinant soluble form of the naturally occurring IL-1 receptor and traps/blocks IL-1; canakinumab is a humanized IL-1β antibody

is evidence that pain can further enhance the inflammatory response. Therefore, the management of the child should include analgesic, as well as anti-inflammatory, therapy. Physical and occupational therapy that improve joint and muscle function, stamina, aerobic capabilities and protect joints may have a direct analgesic benefit. Cognitive behavioral therapy also can decrease pain and improve function.

TABLE 2.2 Major immunomodulatory drugs used in pediatric rheumatology targeting cells

Drug type	Mode of action
High-dose IV steroids	Depletes lymphocyte numbers; blocks cell signaling
Cyclophosphamide	Depletes lymphocytes, B and T cells
Cyclosporine A	Blocks transcription of T cell genes
Mycophenolate mofetil	Inhibits B and T cell proliferation
Azathioprine	Inhibits T lymphocytes
Hydroxychloroquine	Inhibits phospholipid function and binds DNA
Sulfasalazine	Unclear
Leflunomide	Unclear
Colchicine	Inhibits cytoskeletal transport and inflammasome activation
Thalidomide	Inhibits T cell proliferation
Monoclonal antibodies to B cells	Depletes pre- and mature B cell numbers (anti-CD20/rituximab)
Abatacept	Prevents co-stimulation of T cells via blocking CD80/86 and CD28 interaction

A multidisciplinary approach that takes a more functional approach to the child's ability to cope in the home, school and local community may be necessary [7].

2.4 Multidisciplinary Approach to Management

The pediatric rheumatologist leads a team of physicians and allied health professionals in treating children with rheumatic diseases. Others commonly involved in the care of these diseases include ophthalmologists, dentists, orthopedists, podiatrists and rehabilitation specialists and other physicians who care for specific systems involved in these diseases. Rheumatologic clinical nurses and nurse practitioners play an important role in patient education and contact.

The restoration of function is an overlap area between the physical therapist, occupational therapist and rehabilitation physician. There are principles specific to the physical and occupational therapy in inflammatory joint disease as opposed to musculoskeletal rehabilitation after injury or surgery. Inflammation causes weakening and wasting of muscle directly through the inflammatory cytokines, as well as through reflex inhibition from joint swelling and pain. In juvenile dermatomyositis, there is, additionally, inflammation of the skeletal muscles. Joint contractures frequently result. In scleroderma, fibrosis of skin and soft tissues can cause disabling contractures without the synovia being affected. Bone development is affected by inflammation and osteoporosis can occur locally, as well as globally. The biomechanics of complex joints, such as the knee, are particularly easily deranged during inflammatory disease. Specialist physical therapy recommendations are critical during the inflammatory and rehabilitation phases.

Clinical and educational psychologists help with the evaluation and treatment of family dynamics and school re-entry issues as well as issues of coping with chronic disease and treatment adherence. Dieticians aid in the development of a nutrition plan to maximize growth and prevent failure to thrive related to loss of appetite and pain from chronic disease, medications and arthritis. Social workers help obtain necessary community and governmental (or insurance company) support.

2.5   Complementary and Alternative Therapies

The multidisciplinary approach to address all the needs of the child with a rheumatologic problem has already been stressed. Complementary therapies, although few formal trials have been conducted, may be useful for individual children [8]. Relaxation techniques, massage, aromatherapy and acupuncture may help to control pain and should not be discouraged.

Homeopathy is a frequently used remedy. Since the remedies consist of extremely diluted substances, often diluted beyond Avogadro's number, they generally have no untoward effects but the cost and burden of administration, since frequently multiple preparations are given multiple times a day, needs to be circumspectly assessed.

There has been an explosion of public interest in oriental and folk remedies. Certain traditional medications have active components similar to the drugs used in the western world, but have not undergone controlled trials. Uninformed use may lead to significant side effects, such as heavy metal nephropathy, bone marrow suppression from alkaloids, and a host of steroid side effects. Others, like echinacea, are considered immunostimulants and in autoimmune conditions should be used with caution. Some may be helpful as in the fish oils, mainly those that contain omega 3. Glucosamine and chondroitin may be useful in osteoarthritis in adults. However, there may be some effect on bone growth in children and caution should be employed in using these supplements in children.

In cases when the practitioner of alternative medicine claims that these remedies should replace conventional drugs, in the presence of continuing clinical and laboratory signs of inflammation, there should be a clear line drawn in favor of drugs which have been demonstrated to be effective in controlled studies. Likewise, over treatment is common in children with amplified pain syndromes; many complementary therapies can be counterproductive.

References

1. Tucker LB, Cabral DA. Transition of the adolescent patient with rheumatic disease: issues to consider. Rheum Dis Clin North Am. 2007;33:661–72.

2. Ćalasan MB, Wulffraat NM. Methotrexate in juvenile idiopathic arthritis: towards tailor-made treatment. Expert Rev Clin Immunol. 2014;10:843–54.
3. Beukelman T, Patkar NM, Saag KG, et al. 2011 American College of Rheumatology recommendations for the treatment of juvenile idiopathic arthritis: initiation and safety monitoring of therapeutic agents for the treatment of arthritis and systemic features. Arthritis Care Res (Hoboken). 2011;63:465–82.
4. Ringold S, Weiss PF, Beukelman T, et al. American College of Rheumatology. 2013 update of the 2011 American College of Rheumatology recommendations for the treatment of juvenile idiopathic arthritis: recommendations for the medical therapy of children with systemic juvenile idiopathic arthritis and tuberculosis screening among children receiving biologic medications. Arthritis Rheum. 2013;65:2499–512.
5. Bertsias GK, Tektonidou M, Amoura Z, et al. European League Against Rheumatism and European Renal Association-European Dialysis and Transplant Association. Joint European League Against Rheumatism and European Renal Association-European Dialysis and Transplant Association (EULAR/ERA-EDTA) recommendations for the management of adult and paediatric lupus nephritis. Ann Rheum Dis. 2012;71:1771–82.
6. La Hausse de Lalouvière L, Ioannou Y, Fitzgerald M. Neural mechanisms underlying the pain of juvenile idiopathic arthritis. Nat Rev Rheumatol. 2014;10:205–11.
7. Weiss JE, Luca NJ, Boneparth A, Stinson J. Assessment and management of pain in juvenile idiopathic arthritis. Paediatr Drugs. 2014;16:473–81.
8. April KT, Walji R. The state of research on complementary and alternative medicine in pediatric rheumatology. Rheum Dis Clin North Am. 2011;37:85–94.

Chapter 3
Juvenile Idiopathic Arthritis (JIA)

3.1 Introduction

The majority of children with inflammatory rheumatologic conditions have some form of arthritis. The different categories are determined by articular and extra-articular manifestations and it may be months before one is sure of the diagnosis. Not knowing the category does not preclude treatment, but one should always be willing to change the diagnosis as the illness progresses. Juvenile idiopathic arthritis (JIA) is an umbrella term for several distinct arthritides lasting more than 6 weeks with unknown etiology (Table 3.1) [1]. The pathogenesis of these diseases involves both autoimmune and genetic factors. Dysregulation of the immune and inflammatory systems is observed and include increased immune complexes, complement activation and disordered Th1, Th2, and Th17 cell interactions with predominance of Th1 and Th17 cells in the synovium. Additionally, hormonal, infectious and other environmental agents, yet to be identified, are likely involved. The term "juvenile" refers to the onset of arthritis at 16 years of age or younger. However, it is an arbitrary distinction and, as far as we know, there are no biological reasons why nearly all these conditions cannot occur in adults. In fact, several are more common in adults, such as rheumatoid factor (RF) positive polyarthritis and psoriatic arthritis. Conversely, the

R.M. Laxer et al., *Pediatric Rheumatology in Clinical Practice*,
DOI 10.1007/978-3-319-13099-6_3,
© Springer-Verlag London 2016

TABLE 3.1 Juvenile idiopathic arthritis subtypes

Oligoarthritis (persistent and extended)
Polyarthritis rheumatoid factor negative
Polyarthritis rheumatoid factor positive
Systemic
Enthesitis-related arthritis
Psoriatic arthritis
Undifferentiated arthritis

onset of systemic and anti-nuclear antibody (ANA) positive oligoarticular JIA in Caucasians is most commonly below the age of 6 years and these are much less frequent in adults than in the pediatric age group.

3.2   Oligoarthritis

3.2.1   Definition

Arthritis in this group affects four or fewer joints within the first 6 months of disease. If more than four joints become involved after 6 months, it is defined as extended oligoarthritis, otherwise it is known as persistent oligoarthritis [1].

3.2.2   Epidemiology

This is the most common form of JIA and preferentially afflicts 1 to 3-year-old Caucasian girls. Although all races can be affected, the prevalence is much reduced in non-Caucasians. Girls outnumber boys 4:1. It affects about 60 per 100,000 children.

3.2.3   Etiology

About 70 % of oligoarticular JIA patients have ANA and there is a disproportionate number with the HLA alleles at DRB1*08 locus [2]. Other factors may be at play, giving rise to the predominance of girls.

3.2.4   Clinical Manifestations

Approximately half of oligoarticular JIA patients will have a single joint involved at onset, mainly the knee (Fig. 3.1). The next most commonly affected joint is the ankle (Fig. 3.2). Small joints of the hand are the third most commonly affected, and may portend the later onset of psoriatic arthritis [3]. Temporomandibular joint (TMJ) arthritis is not uncommon, but is often detected late in the course of the disease, as symptoms are not common. Initial wrist involvement is rare and may indicate the progression to extended oligoarthritis. Shoulders and hips are almost never involved. Cervical spine disease, while rare, may be manifest by torticollis. Uveitis is rarely a presenting sign. It may be manifested clinically by an

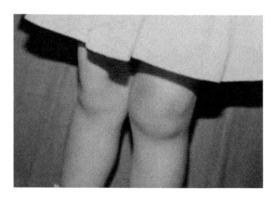

FIGURE 3.1   Unilateral arthritis of the left knee in oligoarticular JIA

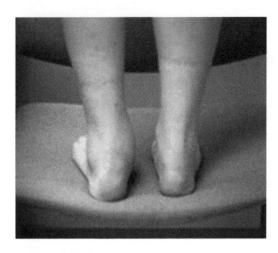

FIGURE 3.2 Posterior view of unilateral arthritis of the left ankle, showing valgus deformity of the hind foot

irregular pupil. The anterior uveitis (iridocyclitis or iritis) may be low grade and early inflammation is only detectable by slit lamp examination.

Most children will complain of joint pain, morning stiffness and gelling and a parent will notice a limp and joint swelling. However, 25 % of children report no pain and swelling is the only abnormality.

The most common extra-articular manifestation is uveitis. In oligoarthritis up to 20 % of patients can develop uveitis, which is usually asymptomatic. The eye is neither red nor photophobic. It is more prevalent in the children who are ANA positive. The astute physician should look for keratopunctate deposits on the cornea, pupillary irregularity or synechiae at presentation (Fig. 3.3) and, if present, should send the child immediately for an ophthalmologic consultation; if absent, the child should have a slit lamp examination of the eyes every 3–4 months for the first year regardless. Some physicians will decrease the surveillance to every 6 months if the ANA is negative, since a positive ANA test is a strong predictor of uveitis (Table 3.2) [4].

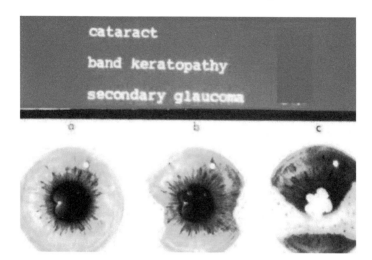

FIGURE 3.3 Complications of uveitis of JIA. *Left to right*: Cataract, synechiae, band keratopathy. Late outcome is secondary glaucoma

3.2.5 Laboratory Features

The most common abnormal finding is a positive ANA test. It is present in 50–70 % of children with oligoarthritis. Occasionally, the child will have elevated acute phase reactants, such as an elevated ESR or CRP, but these are usually mildly elevated. Greatly elevated acute phase reactants may be associated with subclinical inflammatory bowel disease or malignancy. The blood counts are usually normal and the RF is negative.

3.2.6 Establishing the Diagnosis

The diagnosis is made by the presence of chronic arthritis (longer than 6 weeks) in four or fewer joints in the first 6 months of disease and the absence of other causes.

Exclusions to oligoarthritis include psoriasis in a first -degree relative, HLA-B27 associated disease in a first-

TABLE 3.2 Recommended frequency of slit lamp examination to check for asymptomatic uveitis for children with JIA

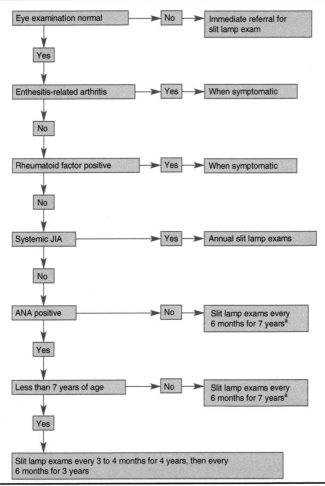

[a]Some physicians will have these children get a slit lamp examination every 3–4 months initially for 1–2 years since it is possible for children with a negative ANA test to develop uveitis. After 7 years, eye exams can be annual. If uveitis develops, then this scheme does not apply, and the frequency of slit lamp exams will be more frequent as per the ophthalmologist

degree relative, systemic JIA, a positive RF test, or a positive HLA-B27 test in a boy aged 6 years or older. Table 3.3 is a general outline to assist in the diagnosis of children with various forms of JIA.

The differential diagnosis is broadest in monoarticular arthritis and includes septic arthritis, reactive arthritis, foreign body synovitis, pigmented villonodular synovitis, arterial-venous malformation, bleeding disorders (such as hemophilia), or severe trauma, including non-accidental trauma (Chap. 1, Table 1.3). Routine trauma, such as from a fall, does not cause persistent joint swelling and trauma is very rarely a cause of joint swelling unless there is an internal derangement seen in older, not younger, children. Lyme disease (in an endemic area) frequently causes knee swelling usually for less than 6 weeks, although it is frequently recurrent. Leukemia can cause limb pain and may be associated with swelling, but frequently is associated with systemic manifestations and more pain and disability than in children with JIA [5].

3.2.7   Treatment

The initial treatment should be corticosteroid intra-articular injection. Triamcinolone hexacetonide is the preferred agent although triamcinolone acetonide may be used if the former is unavailable. For a knee, we use 1 mg/kg of triamcinolone hexacetonide and 2 mg/kg of triamcinolone acetonide (up to 60 mg and 120 mg respectively). The duration of benefit is highly variable (Table 3.4) [6]. Non-steroidal anti-inflammatory drugs (NSAIDs) may help control symptoms, but they do not alter the natural history. If the arthritis recurs, joint injections can be repeated up to three times in a 12-month period. The response to a second joint injection is not predicted by the response of the first. However, if it is resistant to multiple injections, then a disease-modifying agent, such as methotrexate, leflunomide or an anti-TNF agent should be used, especially if extended disease has developed. Some physicians would

TABLE 3.3 Algorithm for the diagnosis of JIA[a]

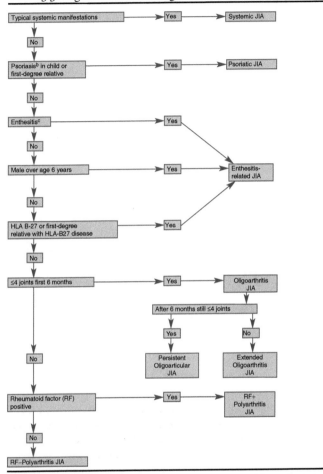

[a]These are general guidelines, since there are specific exclusions not fully outlined. A few children will qualify as having either none or two forms of JIA and are, therefore, classified as having undifferentiated JIA. The arthritis is defined in the ILAR classification as occurring in a child of 16 or under, and persisting for over 6 weeks
[b]Psoriasis confirmed by a physician
[c]Number and site of tender entheses are not specified but we prefer at least three sites other than metatarsal heads

TABLE 3.4 A treatment algorithm for persistent oligoarticular JIA and oligoarticular psoriatic JIA[a]

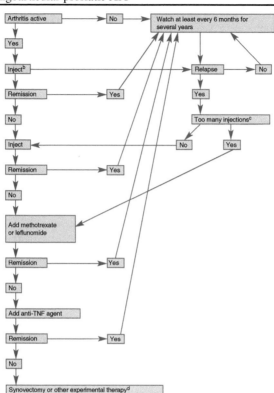

[a]NSAIDs are used for symptomatic care, such as morning stiffness or musculoskeletal pain. They are withdrawn once remission is achieved. Physical and occupational therapies are used as needed

[b]Methotrexate and subsequent agents, if needed, are added at the time of first injection of the temporomandibular joint, due to the inaccessibility of monitoring recurrent arthritis. Midfoot arthritis may also be an indication for more early addition of methotrexate and subsequent agents

[c]The number of acceptable total injections and injections per year has not been strictly defined and will vary depending on the patient, joint, and physician. If a single joint requires more than three injections in a 12-month period, it is recommended to add a disease modifying anti-rheumatic drug (DMARD)

[d]In psoriatic arthritis anti-IL-23 and IL-17 and phosphodiesterase 4 inhibitors show promise

add a disease modifying agent at the time of an injection of the temporomandibular joint, since these are particularly prone to destruction. In addition, they are important for function and are hard to evaluate clinically once disease has been established.

A few children will have persistent flexion contractures that will require physiotherapy. Besides exercise and stretching, night splints and serial casting are occasionally required. Serial casting is done two or three times a week for up to a month. Some children with leg length discrepancy (resulting from overgrowth of the affected knee) may require a shoe lift/raise. Uveitis is usually controlled with topical medications, but if it is resistant or side effects develop, methotrexate, and anti-TNF agents, have been shown to help [7]. Other medications such as cyclosporine, tacrolimus, mycophenolate mofetil and abatacept may also have a role in uveitis should methotrexate fail.

3.2.8   Outcome

Most children with oligoarthritis do well and the disease will remit in as many as 65 % of children over the years for the persistent oligoarthritic subgroup [8]. Extended oligoarthritis occurs in about 30 % and the outcome was poor until methotrexate was introduced as the treatment of choice. Remission is induced in 60–70 % while on methotrexate. Anti-TNF agents are effective if patients fail to respond fully to methotrexate, especially if given in combination with methotrexate. The worst outcome is visual loss, which is more frequent in children with significant eye involvement at the time of their first ophthalmologic visit. Other sequelae include leg length discrepancy in those with knee arthritis. Persistent swelling and pain also lead to muscle atrophy. Thigh atrophy in children with knee arthritis is often permanent.

3.3   Polyarthritis, Rheumatoid Factor (RF) Negative

3.3.1   Definition

Arthritis affecting five or more joints in the first 6 months of the disease and a negative RF test [1].

3.3.2   Epidemiology

This form of JIA also preferentially afflicts 1–3 year old Caucasian girls, although all races can be affected. Girls outnumber boys 3:1. It affects about 40 per 100,000 children.

3.3.3   Etiology

The cause is unknown, but about 40 % have ANA.

3.3.4   Clinical Manifestations

The arthritis is usually insidious and symmetrical, frequently involving the small joints, including the distal interphalangeal joints. Children with less than 10 inflamed joints behave more frequently like those with oligoarthritis than those with widespread arthritis. Uveitis occurs in 10–20 %, generally those with relatively few affected joints.

3.3.5   Laboratory Features

Polyarthritis may be associated with elevated acute phase reactants and mild anemia. The ANA test is positive in up to 40 % and RF is negative by definition.

3.3.6 Establishing the Diagnosis

The diagnosis requires arthritis to be present in five or more joints for at least 6 weeks. The RF test has to be negative (Table 3.3). Other major diagnostic considerations include autoimmune connective tissue diseases (particularly in the older girl who is ANA positive), lymphoma, leukemia, or prolonged viral synovitis.

3.3.7 Treatment

Children with polyarthritis generally require a disease-modifying agent at the time of diagnosis, or shortly after the diagnosis is firmly established (Table 3.5). If, within several months methotrexate is not working well enough, or is not tolerated, an anti-TNF agent (etanercept, adalimumab or infliximab) is indicated [9]. The use of leflunomide is also an option before starting an anti-TNF agent. The role of early combination therapy including methotrexate and anti-TNF agents is not fully clarified. Abatacept and tocilizumab are alternatives to anti-TNF agents. Some children require multiple joint injections to maintain control of the arthritis and function, as well as physical and occupational therapy.

3.3.8 Outcome

Approximately 40–50 % (or less) of children will go into long-term remission, but usually only after years [8]. As a result, if untreated, there may be significant physical and psychological sequelae. Children without hip and shoulder arthritis do better and rarely become significantly disabled.

TABLE 3.5 A treatment algorithm for polyarthritis course JIA with disease modifying agents

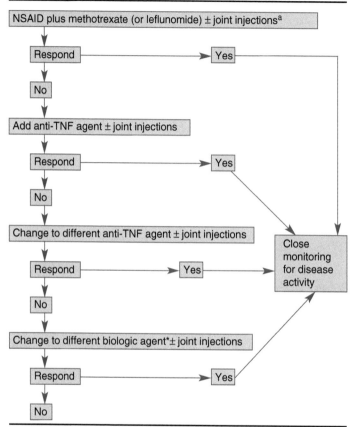

[a]NSAIDs are used for symptomatic care, such as morning stiffness or musculoskeletal pain. They are withdrawn once remission is achieved. Temporomandibular joint and hip arthritis should be injected early on, due to the importance of these joints to function. Physical and occupational therapies are used as needed. * Biologic agents may include abatacept, rituximab, tocilizumab, or tofacitinib

3.4   Polyarthritis, Rheumatoid Factor (RF) Positive

3.4.1   Definition

Arthritis which affects five or more joints in the first 6 months of disease and a positive RF tests on two occasions at least 3 months apart [1].

3.4.2   Epidemiology

This form of JIA is more typically seen in adolescent girls. It affects about 10 per 100,000 children.

3.4.3   Etiology

The cause is unknown, but it is associated with HLA-DR4, as in adult rheumatoid arthritis.

3.4.4   Clinical Manifestations

The arthritis is usually insidious and symmetrical, frequently involving the small joints of the hands, typically the PIP joints and wrists. At onset low grade fever may be present, but it is distinctly different from systemic JIA. Children may have hard, non-tender nodules, predominately on extensor surfaces. Felty syndrome (splenomegaly and neutropenia) and vasculitis rarely occurs in untreated childhood RF+ polyarthritis. Uveitis does not occur in this onset type.

3.4.5   Laboratory Features

Polyarthritis may be associated with elevated acute phase reactants and anemia. The ANA test is often positive and (by definition) the RF is positive on two occasions 3 months apart. In these patients, anti-cyclic citrullinated peptide antibodies (anti-CCP) may be more specific and portend destructive arthritis [10].

3.4.6   Establishing the Diagnosis

The diagnosis requires arthritis to be present in five or more joints for at least 6 weeks. The RF test has to be positive on two different occasions 3 months apart (Table 3.3). Most other diagnostic considerations (viral infections, neoplasms, systemic lupus and other autoimmune diseases) are eliminated by the time the RF test is repeated and positive again.

3.4.7   Treatment

Children with RF positive polyarthritis are at high risk for prolonged erosive arthritis and require a disease-modifying agent as soon as possible (Table 3.5). Anti-TNF agents should be added if methotrexate is not adequately controlling the arthritis, since they have been shown to prevent bony erosions, especially in combination with methotrexate. Abatacept and tocilizumab are alternatives to anti-TNF agents. Although not studied formally in children, rituximab may be beneficial in this type of arthritis. Some children require multiple joint injections and/or short courses of low-dose corticosteroids to maintain control of the arthritis and function and usually require physical and occupational therapy.

3.4.8   Outcome

Children with RF positive polyarthritis have long lasting disease that usually requires ongoing treatment. If controlled, the functional outcome can be quite good [8]. However, there are children who do not respond and will have joint deformity and permanent dysfunction.

3.5   Systemic JIA (sJIA)

3.5.1   Definition

Arthritis with quotidian spiking fevers of $\geq 39°$ C for more than 2 weeks, accompanied by at least one of the following: an evanescent rash, lymphadenopathy, serositis, or hepatosplenomegaly. The rheumatoid factor test is negative [1].

3.5.2   Epidemiology

This occurs in young children with median age of onset, in most series, at around 4 years of age. The incidence is the same in both sexes in Caucasians, unlike the other types of JIA. The prevalence of sJIA is about 10 cases per 100,000, although some surveys have suggested that it may be more frequent in Japan and India.

3.5.3   Etiology

Unlike other types of arthritis, sJIA is primarily an autoinflammatory disease involving activation of the innate immune system. Recently an association between HLA-DRB1*11 and sJIA was reported and non-HLA genes, such as macrophage migration inhibitory factor (MIF) and interferon regulatory factor (IRF), have been shown to be associated with JIA as a whole and a variant of the interleukin-6 (IL-6) gene confers susceptibility [11]. These genes predispose the patient to a vigorous inflammatory response to stimuli, such as infectious agents, and the net effect of the interaction between pro and anti-inflammatory proteins is probably the key to the clinical features in this subtype of JIA.

3.5.4   Clinical Manifestations

The fever is typically spiking in character with a peak of at least 39° C (Fig. 3.4). It occurs once or twice a day and recurs daily. This is accompanied by an evanescent salmon pink macular/urticarial rash (Fig. 3.5). The macular rash may occasionally be itchy. The child is usually unwell and irritable during the fever, but often recovers in between. Other accompanying symptoms are headache (sometimes with signs of meningitis), arthralgia or arthritis, myalgia,

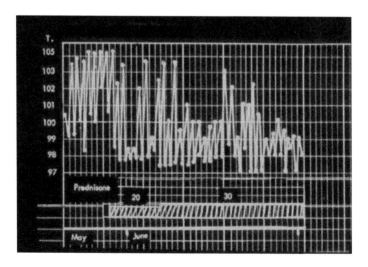

FIGURE 3.4 Daily spiking fever of systemic JIA, despite high-dose prednisolone (>2 mg/kg) in a 5-year-old

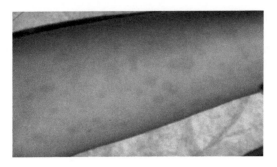

Figure 3.5 Typical rash of systemic JIA, which is centripetal in distribution and evanescent

abdominal pain from serositis that can mimic an acute abdomen, breathlessness and chest pain on lying flat indicating pericarditis, as well as acute chest pain from pleuritis. There is a wide variation in the severity of symptoms, ranging from fever and rash for 2–3 weeks followed by mild arthritis, to simultaneous onset of all the symptoms described above. In the most severe cases, they may also present with features of macrophage activation syndrome – MAS (also known as secondary hemophagocytic lymphohistiocytosis (HLH)), with anemia, jaundice, purpura, liver dysfunction and encephalopathy in the later stages [12].

3.5.5   Laboratory Features

There are no specific tests for sJIA, but there are characteristic patterns of laboratory abnormalities. There is typically a very high CRP, ESR, neutrophilia, thrombocytosis and anemia, which may be profound. Liver enzymes and coagulation screen (especially D-Dimer) may be abnormal in the more severe cases and certainly in MAS. Ferritin levels are often markedly elevated, especially in MAS. There are no autoantibodies or rheumatoid factor detected and complement levels are normal or high (as acute phase reactants) [13].

3.5.6   Establishing a Diagnosis

There are many illnesses in young children that can mimic sJIA (Table 3.6). Apart from arthritis, the fever is classic and an accurate fever chart will often help eliminate some of the differential diagnoses. The rash is like a viral exanthem, but the difference is that it is evanescent. If these criteria are not fulfilled unequivocally, it is necessary to screen for infectious agents, urinary vanillomandelic acids and a bone marrow aspirate to exclude infection, neuroblastoma and leukemia respectively. Some physicians do these tests routinely, since malignancies are often close mimics in the early stages of

TABLE 3.6 Differential diagnoses of systemic JIA (sJIA)

Condition	Differentiating features from sJIA
Infections	Positive cultures/serologic tests, continuous fever and rash
Leukemia	Nonquotidian fevers, bone and night pain, constantly systemically unwell, purpura, elevated uric acid and lactate dehydrogenase levels
Neuroblastoma	Nonquotidian fevers, constantly systemically unwell
NOMID/CINCA	Fixed rash, undulating fevers, neurologic complications, bone abnormalities
Kawasaki disease	Fixed rash, mucocutaneous symptoms, coronary artery dilatation and aneurysms
Other primary vasculitis	Undulating fevers, fixed and painful rashes or purpura, systemically ill constantly, renal involvement
SLE	Constant fevers, positive ANA and specific autoantibodies, low complement levels, low CRP, cytopenias, other organs involved

NOMID neonatal onset multisystem inflammatory disease, *CINCA* chronic infantile neurologic cutaneous and articular syndrome, *SLE* systemic lupus erythematosus sJIA [5]. The autoinflammatory syndromes (see Chap. 8) are often mistaken for sJIA, but the character of the fevers and the fixed rashes associated with these syndromes should alert the clinician to a different diagnosis.

3.5.7   Treatment

Mild sJIA often needs nothing more than NSAIDs given to cover the whole 24-h period. Indomethacin is particular helpful for fever and pericarditis. In most cases, however, additional treatment is needed, and drugs of choice are dictated by the degree of activity, severity, and whether the major indication for treatment is arthritis, systemic features, or both. For systemic disease, newer biologics blocking IL-6 (tocilizumab) and IL-1 signaling (anakinra, canakinumab, rilonacept) are highly effective [13, 14]. In fact, they may replace the need for systemic corticosteroids; however, if biologics are not available, systemic corticosteroids are often required. For arthritis, the traditional DMARDs such as methotrexate are not as effective as they are for other forms of JIA; the same holds true for the anti-TNF agents. MAS in sJIA is usually effectively treated with cyclosporine A accompanied by parenteral pulse steroids, with or without anakinra and intravenous immunoglobulin. Table 3.7 is an algorithm of a method of treatment of sJIA.

3.5.8   Outcome

sJIA is heterogeneous in severity, disease course and outcome. It can be monocyclic, with remission within several months in maybe half the children. It can relapse and be characterized by flares of systemic features with mild arthritis or it can continue with persistent destructive arthritis, which is usually more prominent after the regression of systemic features [15]. Patients with severe disease can have flares of extra-articular features at any time, and 23–30 % from two large European series had systemic features 10–15 years after onset [16]. Patients at the severe end of the disease spectrum

TABLE 3.7 A treatment algorithm for systemic JIA

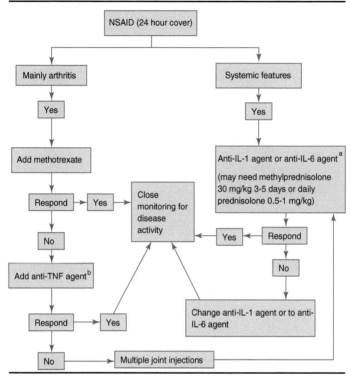

[a]Anakinra, rilonacept, canakinumab, tocilizumab
[b]Etanercept, adalimumab, infliximab

usually have active arthritis into adult life despite standard therapies. Predictors of poor outcome include the presence of systemic features 6 months after onset, thrombocytosis and the presence of polyarthritis with hip involvement [15]. It is likely that the early use of IL-1 and IL-6 inhibitors will substantially improve the prognosis of sJIA.

The incidence of amyloidosis and surgical intervention, such as hip replacements, was much higher in sJIA, and death from amyloidosis in the past used to be 50 %. The mortality rate for sJIA is still higher than the mortality rate associated with other subtypes of JIA in clinical practice now, between

0.6 and 2 %. Causes of mortality are MAS, pulmonary complications, CNS disease and infections related to treatment. As a result of the inadequate control of the disease with the available therapies, growth failure and osteoporosis are serious and lasting complications.

3.6   Enthesitis-Related Arthritis (ERA)

3.6.1   Definition

Arthritis and enthesitis or arthritis or enthesitis with at least two of the following: (1) sacroiliac joint tenderness, or inflammatory lumbosacral pain; (2) HLA-B27 positive; (3) first-degree relative with medically confirmed HLA-B27 associated disease; (4) anterior iridocyclitis, usually symptomatic; and (5) onset of arthritis in a boy 6 years or older [1].

3.6.2   Epidemiology

This form of JIA is more frequent in boys, although it may be under-recognized in symptomatic girls who can have milder disease. The onset typically occurs in children over six and there is a familial predilection. It may be as common as 50 per 100,000 children.

3.6.3   Etiology

ERA is generally thought to be a form of spondyloarthropathy and is usually associated with HLA-B27. In patients who have the HLA-B27 gene, molecular mimicry is thought to play a role, especially regarding Klebsiella and arthritis following infections with Salmonella, Shigella, Campylobacter, Yersinia, Chlamydia, Mycoplasma, Clostridia, or even Giardia.

3.6.4   Clinical Manifestations

The defining feature of this condition is the presence of enthesitis [17]. Enthesitis is inflammation of the tendons and ligaments where they attach to bone (the enthesis) (Fig. 3.6).

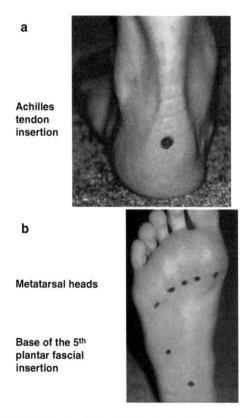

a

**Achilles
tendon
insertion**

b

Metatarsal heads

**Base of the 5th
plantar fascial
insertion**

FIGURE 3.6 (**a**) Enthesis of the Achilles tendon insertion, where pain is often present in enthesitis-related arthritis. (**b**) Entheses of the various tendon and fascial insertions of the foot: Plantar fasciitis or heel pain is a frequent symptom of enthesitis-related arthritis. Achilles tendon insertion (**a**). Metatarsal heads. Base of the 5th plantar fascial insertion (**b**)

Not all entheses are equally significant in ERA and some are prone to mechanical damage, such as in Osgood–Schlatter and Sinding–Larsen–Johansson Syndrome (Chap. 12). Metatarsalgia is not uncommon in children and should not count as enthesitis. One study suggests that pathologic enthesitis be defined as the presence of three of eight sites tested tender to palpation with about 3–4 kg of digital pressure [18]. These sites are: the SI joint, inferior pole of the patella, the Achilles tendon and plantar fascia insertions into the calcaneus. Others have included the medial and lateral epicondyles [19]. Care needs to be taken in establishing the presence of enthesitis.

3.6.5   Investigations

There is no defining laboratory test, although the presence of HLA-B27 is common and helps establish this diagnosis. Some children will have a very high ESR or anemia leading to the suspicion that they may have subclinical inflammatory bowel disease. Doppler ultrasound can identify the inflammation of enthesitis [19].

3.6.6   Establishing a Diagnosis

The diagnosis requires enthesitis or asymmetrical arthritis of the large joints of the lower limbs. Enthesitis or asymmetrical arthritis affects mainly pre-teen and teenage boys. SI joint and spinal inflammation occur in a minority of children with ERA from about 11 years of age on (Table 3.3). A classical symptom of SI joint inflammation is buttock pain with early morning stiffness that improves with activity. Early onset of inflammatory spinal pain usually occurs in the thoracolumbar junction with stiffness and pain after rest that improves with activity. Exclusions from the diagnosis include systemic features of sJIA, a positive rheumatoid factor, psoriasis or the presence of psoriasis in a first-degree relative.

ERA overlaps with a group of conditions collectively known as spondyloarthropathies, such as ankylosing spondylitis (AS). AS may be heralded by enthesitis. There are several criteria for AS (Table 3.8) and young people with AS frequently, but not always, satisfy the criteria for ERA. Likewise, children who satisfy the criteria for the European Spondylarthropathy Study Group (ESSG) (Table 3.9) could be classified as having ERA, although psoriasis is part of the ESSG criteria and is excluded in ERA [20]. Reactive arthritis usually occurs 2–4 weeks after an infection, is more frequent in children below the age of 10 and typically lasts less than 6 weeks.

There are few conditions that mimic ERA, although children with widespread amplified musculoskeletal pain (see Chap. 12) frequently have very tender entheses that may be mistaken for enthesitis.

TABLE 3.8 New York criteria for ankylosing spondylitis (AS)

Clinical criteria
Limitation of lumbar motion in all 3 planes
History or the presence of pain in the lumbar spine
<2.5 cm of chest excursion at the 4th intercostal space
Definite AS
Grade 3–4 (moderate to ankylosed) bilateral sacroiliac changes on radiograph and at least 1 clinical criterion
Grade 3–4 unilateral or grade 2 (minimal) bilateral sacroiliac changes on radiograph with criterion 1 or criteria 2 and 3
Probable AS
Grade 3–4 bilateral sacroiliac changes on radiograph without clinical criteria

TABLE 3.9 Classification criteria of the European Spondylar-thropathy Study Group (ESSG)

Inflammatory spinal pain[a]

Or

Synovitis (asymmetric or predominantly in the lower extremities)

Plus

One of the following:

> Enthesopathy
>
> Sacroiliitis
>
> Alternating buttock pain
>
> Family history of spondylarthropathy
>
> Inflammatory bowel disease
>
> Psoriasis
>
> Urethritis, cervicitis, or diarrhea within 1 month before the onset of arthritis

[a]Inflammatory spinal pain is defined as pain that is worse with rest, frequently morning stiffness that improves with activity

3.6.7   Treatment

Treatment of arthritis in ERA is similar to oligoarthritis and polyarthritis. Most patients respond to intra-articular corticosteroid injections and many will need sulfasalazine, or methotrexate, along with physiotherapy. If severe, a course of oral corticosteroids is often helpful. Children with enthesitis will generally require a NSAID for symptomatic relief. We empirically favor certain NSAIDs for enthesitis, specifically diclofenac, indomethacin and piroxicam. The aim of treatment is for functional relief since 100 % relief is usually not attained. Occasionally corticosteroid injection of the plantar fascial insertion on the calcaneus is helpful, or for a limited time, oral steroids. Physiotherapy as well as shoe modification can help greatly.

These measures have not proved to significantly modify the course of disease, in particular, axial inflammation. The anti-TNF agents have been shown to be effective agents for axial disease [20, 21]. Anti-TNF agents should be used early in the course of axial disease, before irreversible damage from spinal erosion and fusion occurs [22]. Anti-TNF agents are also associated with dramatic improvement in peripheral arthritis and enthesitis. New therapies in adults, including inhibitors of IL-12/23 and IL-17, have not yet been tested in children.

3.6.8   Outcome

The long-term outcome is unknown. Enthesitis is more symptomatic in teens and young adults, and it tends to improve with age. Boys with HLA-B27 and hip arthritis, or tarsal inflammation (tarsitis), are at high risk of developing progressive spinal involvement. In Mexico, the vast majority of boys with tarsitis later developed AS.

3.7   Psoriatic Arthritis

3.7.1   Definition

Arthritis and psoriasis, or arthritis and at least two of the following: (1) dactylitis, (2) nail abnormalities (two or more nail pits, or onycholysis), or (3) family history of psoriasis in a first-degree relative [1].

3.7.2   Epidemiology

Psoriasis occurs in approximately 2 % of the population and about a quarter of these have arthritis. It is estimated that psoriatic arthritis affects 15 per 100,000 children. In the United States, it is much more common in Caucasians than other racial groups; approximately 90 % of patients are Caucasian. Girls are affected slightly more often than boys. There is a bimodal age of onset between 1 and 3 years of age and 7–10 years, with psoriasis typically occurring within 2 years of the onset of arthritis, although it can follow the arthritis by decades.

3.7.3   Etiology

The cause is unknown, but there is a strong genetic component with 40 % of patients with psoriasis having a relative affected and several candidate genes have been identified and many are HLA- DRB1*08 positive, similar to oligoarthritis JIA.

3.7.4   Clinical Manifestations

There are a host of manifestations that span oligoarthritis and polyarthritis onsets and are similar to spondyloarthropathy [23]. Typically the arthritis is asymmetric, involves both large and small joints, and the total number of joints is limited. It is associated with asymptomatic iridocyclitis in 15 % of children. These features are typical of oligoarthritis and many children are first classified as having oligoarthritis JIA before psoriasis is manifest in the child or relative. Children with small joint involvement of the hand tend to develop psoriatic arthritis, nearly one-third have DIP joint involvement and up to half have dactylitis (Fig. 3.7). Children with HLA-B27 develop axial disease similar to ankylosing spondylitis. Rarely, arthritis mutilans occurs with marked joint destruction.

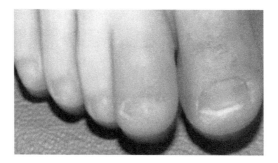

Figure 3.7 Dactylitis of the second toe in psoriatic arthritis, with accompanying nail dystrophy in the first toe

3.7.5 Laboratory Features

The ANA test is positive in up to half of the children with psoriatic arthritis. By definition the RF is negative.

3.7.6 Establishing the Diagnosis

The diagnosis is best established when a child with chronic arthritis has psoriasis. Nail changes (i.e., multiple nail pits), dactylitis, or psoriasis in a first-degree relative are supportive (Table 3.3). Exclusions include positive rheumatoid factor, HLA-B27 disease in first-degree relatives of the child, or sJIA.

3.7.7 Treatment

The treatment is similar to treatment of oligoarthritis or polyarthritis JIA; intra-articular corticosteroid injections are greatly beneficial for those with limited arthritis (Table 3.4). NSAIDs help with symptoms, such as morning stiffness, but do not alter the long-term outcome. Methotrexate is of great benefit for both psoriasis and arthritis. In children with more aggressive disease, anti-TNF therapy is indicated and may significantly limit bony destruction [24]. Oral corticosteroids are rarely needed and withdrawal of oral steroids may exacerbate the psoriasis. Newer therapies approved in adults (phosphodiesterase and IL-12/23 inhibitors) have not yet been tested in children.

3.7.8   Outcome

Children with psoriatic arthritis tend to have longer lasting disease, and a small but significant percentage (up to 10 %) of untreated patients may be disabled. The iridocyclitis of psoriatic arthritis can, rarely, lead to blindness, so close monitoring is indicated (Table 3.2).

3.7.9   Unclassified Arthritis

Up to 10 % of children with chronic arthritis cannot be classified by the above criteria [25]. This is either because they do not fit a category, or they fit more than one category. Children with undifferentiated JIA are followed with a diagnosis of just chronic arthritis and may eventually become diagnosable, e.g., develop psoriasis, or enthesitis, or a connective tissue disease. Regardless of being classifiable, or not, it is always best to be flexible in our thinking about these diseases and constantly on alert for new manifestations that will change our original diagnosis.

References

1. Petty RE, Southwood TR, Manners P, et al. International League of Associations for Rheumatology classification of juvenile idiopathic arthritis: second revision, Edmonton, 2001. J Rheumatol. 2004;31:390–2.

2. Hollenbach JA, Thompson SD, Bugawan TL, et al. Juvenile idiopathic arthritis and HLA class I and class II interactions and age-at-onset effects. Arthritis Rheum. 2010;62:1781–91.

3. Huemer C, Malleson PN, Cabral DA, et al. Patterns of joint involvement at onset differentiate oligoarticular juvenile psoriatic arthritis from pauciarticular juvenile rheumatoid arthritis. J Rheumatol. 2002;29:1531–5.

4. Cassidy J, Kivlin J, Lindsley C, Nocton J. Ophthalmologic examinations in children with juvenile rheumatoid arthritis. Pediatrics. 2006;117:1843–5.

5. Tamashiro MS, Aikawa NE, Campos LM, et al. Discrimination of acute lymphoblastic leukemia from systemic-onset juvenile idiopathic arthritis at disease onset. Clinics (Sao Paulo). 2011;66:1665–9.

6. Zulian F, Martini G, Gobber D, Agosto C, Gigante C, Zacchello F. Comparison of intra-articular triamcinolone hexacetonide and triamcinolone acetonide in oligoarticular juvenile idiopathic arthritis. Rheumatology (Oxford). 2003;42:1254–9.

7. Hawkins MJ, Dick AD, Lee RJ, et al. Managing juvenile idiopathic arthritis-associated uveitis. Surv Ophthalmol. 2016; 61:197-210.

8. Nordal E, Zak M, Aalto K, et al. Ongoing disease activity and changing categories in a long-term nordic cohort study of juvenile idiopathic arthritis. Arthritis Rheum. 2011;63:2809–18.

9. Gowdie PJ, Tse SM. Juvenile idiopathic arthritis. Pediatr Clin North Am. 2012;59:301–27.

10. Berntson L, Nordal E, Fasth A, et al. Anti-type II collagen antibodies, anti-CCP, IgA RF and IgM RF are associated with joint damage, assessed eight years after onset of juvenile idiopathic arthritis (JIA). Pediatr Rheumatol Online J. 2014;12:22.

11. Ogilvie EM, Fife MS, Thompson SD, et al. The -174G allele of the interleukin-6 gene confers susceptibility to systemic arthritis in children: a multicenter study using simplex and multiplex juvenile idiopathic arthritis families. Arthritis Rheum. 2003;48:3202–6.

12. Behrens EM, Beukelman T, Gallo L, et al. Evaluation of the presentation of systemic onset juvenile rheumatoid arthritis: data from the Pennsylvania Systemic Onset Juvenile Arthritis Registry (PASOJAR). J Rheumatol. 2008;35:343–8.

13. Hay AD, Ilowite NT. Systemic juvenile idiopathic arthritis: a review. Pediatr Ann. 2012;41:e232–7.

14. Bruck N, Schnabel A, Hedrich CM. Current understanding of the pathophysiology of systemic juvenile idiopathic arthritis (sJIA) and target-directed therapeutic approaches. Clin Immunol (Orlando, Fla). 2015;159:72–83.

15. Spiegel LR, Schneider R, Lang BA, et al. Early predictors of poor functional outcome in systemic-onset juvenile rheumatoid arthritis: a multicenter cohort study. Arthritis Rheum. 2000;43:2402–9.

16. Hafner R, Truckenbrodt H. Course and prognosis of systemic juvenile chronic arthritis – retrospective study of 187 patients. Klin Padiatr. 1986;198:401–7.

17. Ramanathan A, Srinivasalu H, Colbert RA. Update on juvenile spondyloarthritis. Rheum Dis Clin North Am. 2013;39:767–88.

18. Sherry DD, Sapp LR. Enthesalgia in childhood: site-specific tenderness in healthy subjects and in patients with seronegative enthesopathic arthropathy. J Rheumatol. 2003;30:1335–40.

19. Chauvin NA, Ho-Fung V, Jaramillo D, Edgar JC, Weiss PF. Ultrasound of the joints and entheses in healthy children. Pediatr Radiol. 2015;45:1344–54.

20. Burgos-Vargas R, Tse SM, et al. A randomized, double-blind, placebo-controlled multicenter study of adalimumab in pediatric patients with enthesitis-related arthritis. Arthritis Care Res (Hoboken). 2015;67:1503–12.

21. Henrickson M, Reiff A. Prolonged efficacy of etanercept in refractory enthesitis-related arthritis. J Rheumatol. 2004;31:2055–61.

22. Gmuca S, Weiss PF. Juvenile spondyloarthritis. Curr Opin Rheumatol. 2015;27:364–72.

23. Butbul Aviel Y, Tyrrell P, Schneider R, et al. Juvenile psoriatic arthritis (JPsA): juvenile arthritis with psoriasis? Pediatr Rheumatol Online J. 2013;11:11.

24. Windschall D, Muller T, Becker I, Horneff G. Safety and efficacy of etanercept in children with the JIA categories extended oligoarthritis, enthesitis-related arthritis and psoriasis arthritis. Clin Rheumatol. 2015;34:61–9.

25. Modesto C, Anton J, Rodriguez B, et al. Incidence and prevalence of juvenile idiopathic arthritis in Catalonia (Spain). Scand J Rheumatol. 2010;39:472–9.

Chapter 4
Systemic Lupus Erythematosus

4.1 Introduction

A prototypic autoimmune disease, systemic lupus erythematosus (SLE) typically presents in adolescent females, but it can occur as early as the first year of life. Recent advances in the management of lupus have improved the outcome tremendously, such that the 10-year-survival rate is now over 90 %. Nevertheless, lupus is associated with significant morbidity from the acute disease related events and treatment side effects (Table 4.1).

4.2 Etiology and Pathogenesis

The etiology of SLE is multifactorial and relates to dysregulation at multiple levels of the immune system. The underlying causes of this dysregulation include complex interactions involving environmental, genetic and endocrine influences. The end result of these interactions is the production of multiple autoantibodies that are both organ-specific and directed against a host of nuclear and cytoplasmic antigens. These antibodies can either target cells directly (e.g. immune cytopenias) or form circulating or in situ immune complexes that deposit in vital organs and recruit complement, inflammatory cells and cytokines, which lead to local inflammation and organ damage.

R.M. Laxer et al., *Pediatric Rheumatology in Clinical Practice*, 63
DOI 10.1007/978-3-319-13099-6_4,
© Springer-Verlag London 2016

Table 4.1 Long-term morbidity in systemic lupus erythematosus

Central nervous system
Cognitive dysfunction
Stroke
Transverse myelitis
Cardiovascular
Premature atherosclerosis
Heart failure
Renal
Hypertension
Dialysis
Transplantation
Skin
Scarring alopecia
Psychologic
Depression
Drug-related
Cyclophosphamide
Infertility
Malignancy
Corticosteroids
Avascular necrosis
Osteoporosis
Obesity following being cushingoid
Striae
Growth failure
Cataracts

That genetics plays an important role is evident by different prevalence figures in different ethnic groups. Lupus is more common in certain ethnic groups (Latino, Asian, and Afro-Caribbean), and strongly associated with HLA haplotypes. Recent genome-wide association studies (GWAS) have demonstrated that over 40 genes contribute to the development of SLE and involve multiple immunologic abnormalities that ultimately lead to autoantibody production. These include defective apoptosis, intrinsic abnormalities of B cells and T cells (number and function) and innate immune system abnormalities which lead both inflammasome activation and excessive interferon production. In addition, genetic disorders associated with complement component deficiencies have been associated with a much higher incidence of SLE and lupus-like disease.

4.3 Epidemiology

Lupus is most common in women of child bearing age. The incidence peaks between 19 and 29 years of age. Approximately 10–20 % of cases begin in childhood. Incidence rates have varied between 0.36 and 2.5 per 100,000; differences likely relate to ethnicity, access to care and study methodology. Wide differences in prevalence have also been reported, from approximately 2–25 per 100,000 individuals [1]. In the Lupus Clinic at The Hospital for Sick Children (Toronto, Ontario, Canada), girls outnumber boys 5:1 [2], but this increases to 10–20 women to 1 man in adulthood.

4.4 Clinical Manifestations

The clinical manifestations reflect the degree of systemic inflammation as well as the organ system(s) affected. Systemic manifestations, both at the time of diagnosis as well as at a time of disease exacerbations, frequently include constitutional features such as fever, anorexia, lethargy, weight loss and fatigue. The diagnosis is based on the presence of multi-system involvement with compatible laboratory abnormalities. The presence of 4 of 11 American College of Rheumatology (ACR) Classification Criteria for SLE (with 1997 revision) [3, 4] (see Table 4.2) has both a very high sensitivity and specificity for the diagnosis of pediatric SLE [5]. However, it is important to point out that the published criteria are *classification*, not diagnostic criteria and that SLE can be diagnosed by experienced clinicians in the absence of the required number of classification criteria. A new set of classification criteria, the SLICC criteria (Table 4.3) [6], resulted in fewer misclassifications in a large set of case scenarios compared to the ACR criteria. Major differences are the inclusion of both acute and chronic skin rashes and the addition of hypocomplementemia and direct Coombs test without anemia.

4.4.1   Mucocutaneous

Eruptions of the skin and mucus membranes occur in the majority of patients, usually at presentation, and comprise four of the classification criteria. The "butterfly" or malar rash typically occurs on the cheeks, crosses the bridge of the nose but spares the nasal labial folds (Fig. 4.1). Findings range from mild erythema to an "angry-looking" vasculitic eruption, which is frequently spotty and not always a typical butterfly rash. Oral ulcers typically involve the hard palate and are usually painless (Fig. 4.2). Therefore a careful search for these ulcerations is warranted. Nasal ulcers may also be asymptomatic, but occasionally lead to septum perforation. Discoid lupus lesions typically occur on the scalp, ears or extensor surfaces. They are hyperkeratotic and purplish with follicular plugging. Discoid lesions are unique in that they may leave permanent scarring and alopecia. Rarely a child will have just discoid lupus without systemic disease. Photosensitivity may result in a blistering rash and sun exposure can precipitate disease flares.

TABLE 4.2 The 1982 criteria for classification of systemic lupus erythematosus with 1997 revision [3, 4]

Criterion	Definition
Malar rash	Fixed erythema, flat or raised, over the malar eminences, tending to spare the nasolabial folds
Discoid rash	Erythematous raised patches with adherent keratotic scaling and follicular plugging; atrophic scarring may result in older lesions
Photosensitivity	Skin rash as a result of unusual reaction to sunlight, by patient history or physician observation
Oral ulcers	Oral or nasopharyngeal ulceration, usually painless, observed by physician
Arthritis	Nonerosive arthritis involving 2 or more peripheral joints, characterized by tenderness, swelling, or effusion
Serositis	Pleuritis: convincing history of pleuritic pain or rubbing heard by a physician or evidence of pleural effusion
	Or
	Pericarditis: documented by ECG or rub or evidence of pericardial effusion
Renal disorder	Persistent proteinuria >0.5 g/day (or >3+ if quantitation not performed)
	Or
	Cellular casts: may be red cell, hemoglobin, granular, tubular, or mixed
Neurologic disorder	Seizures in the absence of offending drugs or known metabolic derangements (e.g., uremia, ketoacidosis or electrolyte imbalance)
	Or
	Psychosis in the absence of offending drugs or known metabolic derangements (e.g., uremia: ketoacidosis or electrolyte imbalance)

(continued)

TABLE 4.2 (continued)

Criterion	Definition
Hematological disorder	Hemolytic anemia with reticulocytosis
	Or
	Leukopenia <4,000/mm^3 total, on two or more occasions
	Or
	Lymphopenia <1,500/mm^3 total, on two or more occasions
	Or
	Thrombocytopenia <100,000/mm^3 total, in the absence of offending drugs
Immunological disorder	Anti-DNA antibody to native DNA in abnormal titer
	Or
	Presence of anti-Sm nuclear antigen
	Or
	Positive finding of antiphospholipid antibody based on an abnormal serum level of IgG or IgM anticardiolipin antibodies
	Or
	a positive test for lupus anticoagulant using a standard method
	Or
	on a false-positive serologic test for syphilis known to be positive for at least six months and confirmed by Treponema pallidum immobilization or fluorescent treponemal antibody absorption test
Antinuclear antibody	An abnormal titer of antinuclear antibody by immunofluorescence or an equivalent assay at any point in time and in the absence of drugs known to be associated with drug-induced lupus syndromes

Table 4.3 Systemic Lupus Erythematosus Collaborating Clinic (SLICC) classification criteria for systemic lupus erythematosus [6]

Requirements: ≥4 criteria (at least one clinical and one laboratory criteria OR biopsy-proven lupus nephritis with positive ANA or anti-DNA

Clinical criteria	Immunologic criteria
1. Acute cutaneous lupus*	1. ANA
2. Chronic cutaneous lupus*	2. Anti-DNA
3. Oral or nasal ulcers*	3. Anti-Sm
4. Non-scarring alopecia	4. Antiphospholipid Ab*
5. Arthritis*	5. Low complement (C3, C4, CH50)
6. Serositis*	6. Direct Coombs test (do not count in presence of hemolytic anemia)
7. Renal*	
8. Neurologic*	
9. Hemolytic anemia	
10. Leukopenia*	
11. Thromocytopenia ($<100,000/mm^3$)	

With permission from Wiley
*See reference [6] for descriptors

Additional important mucocutaneous manifestations include peripheral vasculitic changes on the fingers, toes and earlobes (Fig. 4.3), panniculitis and purpura. Antiphospholipid antibodies are associated with livedo reticularis, a lacy, net-like, reticular rash. Raynaud phenomenon occurs in 20 % of patients and rarely leads to peripheral ischemia or fingertip

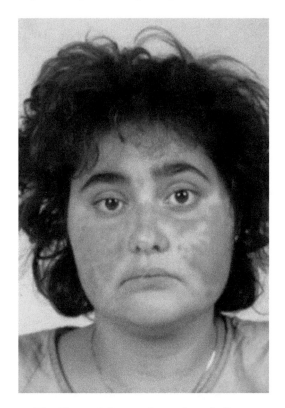

FIGURE 4.1 The "butterfly" or malar rash typically occurs on the cheeks, crosses the bridge of the nose, but spares the nasal labial folds

ulcers. Alopecia may result from discoid lesions or appear spontaneously with generalized hair thinning; a gentle tug on the hair may show how easily the hair falls out.

4.4.2   Musculoskeletal

Arthritis is present in 90 % of patients at some time throughout the course, is often the presenting feature and may be diagnosed as polyarthritis juvenile idiopathic arthritis (JIA)

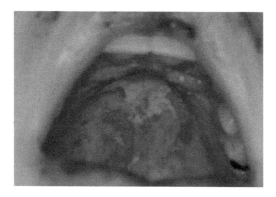

FIGURE 4.2 Oral ulcers typically involve the hard palate and are usually painless

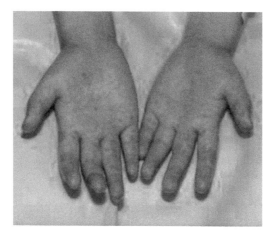

FIGURE 4.3 Vasculitic changes on the fingers of a 4 year old girl with SLE. These lesions also occur frequently on the toes and earlobes

if a careful history, examination and laboratory investigation are not performed. In contrast to the arthritis of JIA, the affected joints are usually less swollen but more painful. While erosive disease does not occur, deformities may result from ligamentous stretching (Jaccoud arthropathy). The combination of active disease and treatment with corticosteroids makes osteopenia a major concern and careful attention to bone health must be paid regarding exercise and diet. Pathologic fractures, particularly vertebral, may result in significant morbidity. Corticosteroids may also lead to avascular necrosis, especially involving the femoral heads, humeral heads and tibial plateaus, causing marked pain and loss of motion. Arthralgias and myalgias are common. Myopathy may occur but is rare. It can occasionally be related to corticosteroid therapy.

4.4.3   Neurologic

The neurologic manifestations listed in the classification criteria are seizures and psychosis, but a host of additional signs and symptoms may occur, as described by the American College of Rheumatology [7] and others [8]. Perhaps the most common is headache; lupus headache may be particularly severe. It is often unrelieved by standard treatment. It may be related to underlying thrombotic disease. Depression is usually reactive to the disease itself, as well as the body altering effect of corticosteroid medications. True psychotic depression may occasionally occur. Stroke may result from large vessel inflammation secondary to vasculitis, thrombosis in the antiphospholipid antibody syndrome, or rarely hemorrhage in patients with severe coagulopathy or severe hypertension. Chorea may be the first manifestation of lupus secondary to antiphospholipid antibodies and may be unilateral. Seizures occur in up to 20 % of patients and may result from hypertension, thrombosis, hemorrhage, vasculitis or antibodies against neuronal cells. Infection also needs to be considered. The recently described posterior reversible encephalopathy syndrome (PRES) has occurred in patients with an acute rise in blood pressure, and usually presents with seizures. Transverse myelitis can occur with the antiphospholipid antibody syndrome or it may be due to arteritis and is potentially fatal.

Recently, there has been increased appreciation of an organic brain syndrome associated with lupus and its treatment. Manifestations can include loss of ability to concentrate, confusion, auditory and more importantly visual hallucinations and even catatonia. This may reflect cerebritis, which results in difficulty processing information, or it may be a late effect from lupus and corticosteroid treatment. Magnetic resonance imaging changes showing cerebral atrophy are common. If due to active disease, the CSF may show increased cells and protein with an increase in the opening pressure on lumbar puncture. Oligoclonal bands, suggesting intrathecal synthesis of immunoglobulins may be present.

Other neurologic manifestations include peripheral neuropathy and myopathy.

4.4.4 Serositis

Pleuritis, manifesting as pleuritic chest pain with or without pleural effusion, is common and may be unilateral or bilateral. Similarly, pericarditis may lead to central chest pain, worse when supine. The combination of serositis, polyarthritis and fever can be confused with the features of systemic-onset JIA. It is critical to look for features of SLE in patients presenting with isolated serositis.

4.4.5 Renal Disease

Renal disease was the major cause of mortality in patients with lupus, but with earlier diagnosis and newer treatment, the outlook for patients with lupus nephritis has improved considerably [9] Immune complex deposits in the kidneys result in a variety of pathologic and clinical manifestations. The International Society of Nephrology/Renal Pathology Society 2003 Classification categorizes lupus nephritis based on the degree of cellular proliferation, extent of glomerular involvement and degree of sclerosis [10]. The histologic abnormalities help determine prognosis and guide treatment.

Importantly, renal disease may transform from one class to another. Immune complex deposits recruit complement, inflammatory cells and cytokines that result in glomerular damage with necrosis and formation of crescents. Tubulo-interstitial inflammation is common. Clinical manifestations of renal disease range from none, to mild hematuria, protein-uria and cellular casts to a clinical picture of nephritic syn-drome with hypertension, edema and renal failure. Rarely, renal vein thrombosis, usually secondary to the presence of antiphospholipid antibodies or severe nephrotic syndrome, may result in acute hematuria and proteinuria with flank pain. Similarly, renal artery thrombi may cause pain second-ary to renal infarction. With current management, less than 10 % of patients develop end-stage renal disease and require dialysis and transplantation. Renal transplantation, when required, should be performed only once the systemic disease is under control. Recurrent renal disease in a transplanted kidney is rare. It is important to keep in mind that not all urinary abnormalities result from active lupus nephritis. For example, urinary tract infections, hematuria from cyclophos-phamide and persistent proteinuria from chronic renal dam-age must be considered and not be treated as a flare of lupus nephritis.

4.4.6   Antiphospholipid Antibody Syndrome (APLS)

Approximately one-third of patients with lupus will develop antiphospholipid antibodies (anticardiolipin, lupus antico-agulant) and some will develop thrombosis. Preliminary clas-sification criteria for APLS have been published [11]. Despite the presence of antibodies that act in the clotting cascade and increase clotting times, patients with APLS form thrombi and both venous and arterial clots may develop.

Common presentations include calf deep vein thrombi, stroke, chorea, livedo reticularis, pulmonary emboli and thrombocytopenia [12]. Recurrent miscarriage with fetal loss is another manifestation. Less common manifestations include Budd-Chiari syndrome, renal and splenic infarcts, and Libman-Sachs endocarditis. Rarely, a catastrophic APLS can develop with widespread clotting. This emergency has a high mortality rate and therefore must be treated immediately and aggressively with high dose corticosteroids, plasmapheresis, anticoagulants and perhaps also IVIG or rituximab. All patients with SLE should be monitored for the presence of these antibodies, and if any clotting occurs, they should probably remain on lifelong anticoagulation. Less commonly, APLS may occur in isolation, without an associated disease (primary APLS).

4.4.7 Hematologic

Disorders of hematologic cellular elements, most commonly from antibodies directed either to the blood components themselves or to stem cells, result in hematocytopenias. Autoimmune thrombocytopenic purpura (AITP) may be a presenting feature of SLE and SLE should be suspected, especially in an older patient with AITP who requires more than standard treatment or has extra-hematologic symptoms with a positive ANA test. Platelet counts may fall to 1–2000/ mm^3. Coombs positive hemolytic anemia may occur alone or in association with AITP (Evans syndrome) and is a possible manifestation of APLS. Both lymphopenia and leukopenia are common. In addition to these lupus-related manifestations, anemia may result from hypersplenism, nutritional deficiency or chronic disease. Thrombocytopenia may be due to APLS. Thrombotic thrombocytopenic purpura in the pediatric population is most commonly related to concurrent SLE or SLE in evolution. Macrophage activation syndrome may occur at presentation or any time during the course of SLE and there must be a high degree of suspicion for its development as early treatment is essential.

4.4.8   Cardiac

In addition to pericarditis, myocarditis may rarely develop, with arrhythmias and ventricular dysfunction, and endocarditis, with noninfectious vegetations on the heart valves (a manifestation of APLS). Premature atherosclerotic heart disease and myocardial infarction occur at young ages in patients with lupus likely related to a combination of active inflammatory disease, coronary artery vasculitis, hypertension, dyslipidemia and long-standing corticosteroid treatment.

4.4.9   Pulmonary

Rarely, pulmonary disease may predominate and can include acute lupus pneumonitis, pulmonary vasculitis with hemorrhage, interstitial fibrosis, pulmonary hypertension and shrinking lung syndrome from diaphragmatic dysfunction. Pulmonary emboli must be suspected in patients with acute respiratory deterioration, especially in patients who are antiphospholipid antibody positive. Finally, pneumonia is not uncommon in immune-compromised patients, with pneumocystis jiroveci being an important organism to consider.

4.4.10   Gastrointestinal

Peritonitis occurs rarely and may be a feature associated with interstitial cystitis. Bowel vasculitis presents with severe abdominal pain and gastrointestinal bleeding. Rarely, pancreatitis is due to lupus and it may also be a side effect of corticosteroids, azathioprine, and mycophenolate mofetil. Hepatic dysfunction with markedly elevated transaminases can be difficult to differentiate from chronic active hepatitis.

4.4.11 Sicca Syndrome

Sicca syndrome, with dry mouth and dry eyes, occurs in about 10 % of pediatric patients with lupus, especially those who have anti-Ro (SS-A) autoantibodies.

4.4.12 Endocrine

Hypothyroidism is the most common endocrine abnormality noted, and anti-thyroid antibodies can occur in up to 40 % of patients. Diabetes is usually secondary to high-dose corticosteroid treatment and therefore is usually transient. Delays in both puberty and growth reflect the impact of both chronic disease and corticosteroid treatment.

4.5 Laboratory Abnormalities

The hallmark of SLE is the presence of autoantibodies, both organ-specific and organ nonspecific. Antinuclear antibodies (ANA) are present in virtually all patients with SLE, so much so that the diagnosis is seriously in doubt in their absence. A positive ANA in a patient suspected of having SLE should promote the search for the specificity of the ANA. Anti-dsDNA antibodies are pathognomonic for SLE and are present in 60 % of cases. Their presence correlates with renal disease. Anti-Sm antibodies are very specific for SLE, but occur in only 25–40 % of cases. They are frequently seen together with anti-RNP. Antibodies to Ro (SS-A) and La (SS-B) are found in about 30 % of patients, and their presence is associated with sicca syndrome (dry mouth and eyes), photosensitivity and risk of neonatal lupus in offspring. Rheumatoid factor, IgM antibodies to IgG, is commonly seen and its presence may lead to a mistaken initial diagnosis of JIA. Hypocomplementemia, usually indicative of complement consumption (or occasionally complement component deficiency) is reflected by reduced levels of C3, C4 and CH50 and correlates with disease activity. Falling levels, that have been previously normal, suggest an impending disease flare and warrant close observation.

All hematologic cell lines may be reduced together or in isolation. Coombs positive hemolytic anemia is characteristic and Coombs test may be positive early on without anemia. Lymphopenia is common and may increase the risk of opportunistic infection. Neutropenia is less common but also predisposes to infection. AITP may be present several years before the patient develops more symptoms.

All other tests (urine, blood chemistries, pulmonary function, cardiac tests, and imaging) reflect the degree of organ involvement. Characteristically, the erythrocyte sedimentation rate is high and the C-reactive protein (CRP) is normal. The CRP will rise with infection, serositis, arthritis and macrophage activation syndrome (in the latter serum ferritin levels will also be markedly increased), but not usually with lupus flares in other organs.

Table 4.4 outline investigation that should be undertaken at onset of disease and during the course of SLE.

4.6   Making the Diagnosis

The key point in making the diagnosis of SLE is to think about it! SLE should be considered in anyone with (1) prolonged marked constitutional symptoms without a diagnosis, (2) multiple organ system disease, (3) polyarthritis in an adolescent, especially a female, (4) unusual presenting features (such as a myocardial infarction in a teenager), (5) hematocytopenias and (6) vasculitic rashes. A thorough history and physical examination, a high index of suspicion and appropriate screening laboratory tests will frequently allow the practitioner to make an early diagnosis.

Other autoimmune diseases, malignancy, and chronic infections may be confused with SLE and must always be considered in the differential diagnosis (see Table 4.5).

TABLE 4.4 Investigations for patients with SLE at onset and during course

System	Tests
General inflammation and indication of flare	CBC, ESR, CRP, C3 and C4 complement
Musculoskeletal	Plain x-rays, bone mineral density, calcium, phosphate, vitamin D, CK (occasionally); MRI if AVN is being considered
Skin	Biopsy (only occasionally required)
Hematologic	CBC and differential, PTT, INR, Coombs, clotting factors (only occasionally required), lupus anticoagulant and anti-phospholipid antibodies
Renal	Urine for microscopy and protein: creatinine ratio, 24 h urine protein collection, serum creatinine, renal biopsy
Neurologic	Brain MRI with gadolinium, MR angiogram and venogram, cerebrospinal fluid analysis with opening pressure, neuropsychiatric testing, EEG for seizures
Immunologic	Antinuclear antibody, anti-DS DNA, anti-Sm, anti-RNP, anti-Ro, anti-La, lupus anticoagulant and anti-phospholipid antibodies

4.7 Treatment

The treatment involves a fine balance between treating the acute events, preventing disease flares, and minimizing treatment-related morbidity. Patients should be seen in a center with experience and expertise in managing childhood SLE. Compliance and lifestyle, especially in adolescents, and the patient and family dynamics are important variables of the treatment plan.

TABLE 4.5 Differential diagnosis of SLE

Disease category	Features in common	Key differentiators
Other connective tissue diseases	Fever, cytopenia, fatigue, rash	Lack of specific autoantibodies (DNA, Sm), specific features unique to specific diseases (e.g., Gottron rash of dermatomyositis)
Malignancy	Fever, cytopenia, fatigue, pain, lymphadenopathy, hepatosplenomegaly	Night pain, bone tenderness, normal complement, no urinary changes
Systemic vasculitis	Fever, fatigue, rash	Nodules, calf pain, positive ANCA, bruits
Juvenile idiopathic arthritis	Arthritis, fatigue, fever, rash, lymphadenopathy, marked anemia	Lack of specific autoantibodies (DNA, Sm), normal or elevated C3, C4, CH50, no major organ dysfunction
Systemic viral infection	Fever, lymphadenopathy, hepatosplenomegaly, cytopenias	Lack of specific autoantibodies (DNA, Sm), normal C3, C4, CH50
Macrophage activation syndrome	Fever, rash, CNS changes, lymphadenopathy, hepatosplenomegaly, cytopenias	Lack of ANA and specific autoantibodies (DNA, Sm), raised CRP, markedly raised ferritin, elevated C3, C4, CH50

The pharmacologic management should be dictated by the degree of organ system involvement. Virtually all patients require systemic corticosteroids, but the dose is dependent upon the disease activity and should be as low as possible to maintain clinical and laboratory control. At times, the laboratory results do not correlate with the clinical manifestations. In general, laboratory tests should not be treated independently of the clinical findings.

Patients with significant cytopenias or CNS disease will require urgent treatment with high-dose corticosteroids, usually at approximately 60 mg/m^2/day (maximum 80 mg/day) with tapering to doses that will keep the disease under control. Many centers use IV methylprednisolone at 30 mg/kg/day (maximum 1 g), often repeated on three consecutive days, to gain control of severe disease, and then maintain improvement with 1–2 mg/kg/day oral prednisolone or its equivalent. Corticosteroids are more effective, but also lead to more side effects, if given in divided doses. The tapering of corticosteroids must be done carefully and an individualized tapering regimen must be developed. Too rapid a taper may lead to disease flare, transient musculoskeletal pain (pseudorheumatism) or pseudotumor cerebri.

Renal and CNS disease almost always require additional agents. Currently, the ideal choice of agent is unclear. Azathioprine, cyclophosphamide and mycophenolate mofetil (MMF) all have their proponents, and varying degrees of evidence for and against. Large studies in adults show that MMF is as effective as cyclophosphamide for the treatment of proliferative lupus nephritis with fewer side effects; the same holds when comparing MMF to azathioprine as maintenance therapy. The Childhood Arthritis and Rheumatology Research Alliance (CARRA) has proposed to study three different treatments in patients with proliferative lupus nephritis [13]. They compare MMF to intravenous cyclophosphamide (each in combination with a tapering corticosteroid regime given primarily orally, intravenously or both). For membranous disease, tacrolimus is preferable. Hypertension and dyslipidemia should be aggressively managed and an ACE inhibitor given to all with any degree of proteinuria, as it seems to decrease the resultant renal damage.

B cell depletion with the monoclonal antibody rituximab has shown encouraging results, especially in patients with cytopenias, but needs further evaluation. Belimumab is a monoclonal antibody that prevents B-cell activation and studies are underway. In adults it is indicated for non-renal lupus mainly as a corticosteroid sparing agent. All patients should be treated with hydroxychloroquine to relieve fatigue, reduce disease flares and rash. It may protect against atherosclerosis and hypercoagulation. Annual ophthalmologic assessment should be done to check for the very rare complication of macular deposition. Musculoskeletal manifestations and serositis may be managed by nonsteroidal anti-inflammatory drugs, hydroxychloroquine or low-dose prednisone. Methotrexate may be useful for persistent arthritis. Topical corticosteroids and topical tacrolimus may help skin disease. All patients should avoid excessive sun exposure and use sunblock. If seizures are isolated they may not require any specific therapeutic intervention. Thrombotic manifestations require appropriate anticoagulation. Osteopenia should be prevented by adequate calcium and vitamin D intake and weight-bearing exercise. Disease related morbidity should be treated in concert with the associated subspecialists.

A general approach to management is listed in Table 4.6.

4.8   Prognosis/Outcome

The outcome of patients with SLE has improved dramatically over the last two decades due to a variety of factors, including: earlier diagnosis and institution of treatment; better use of corticosteroids and immunosuppressive medications; better use of supporting medications and sophisticated critical care units. Nevertheless, while the mortality has been reduced substantially such that the 10-year-survival rate is now greater than 90 %, morbidity remains substantial. SLE is chronic, and while the disease manifestations can generally be well-controlled, there is always the risk of a disease flare. Flares tend to mimic previous disease manifestations. Factors associated with poor outcome include non-adherence to the treatment regime, significant CNS or cardiac disease, and early hypertension with renal disease (Table 4.6).

TABLE 4.6 Treatment of SLE

	Minimalist treatment	May be required	Step up treatment	Occasionally used	Supportive treatment
Skin rash	Avoid sun exposure, sun blocks, topical corticosteroids	Low-dose systemic corticosteroids hydro-xychloroquine	Thalidomide, vitamin A, cyclosporine, topical tacrolimus		Avoid sun exposure, sun blocks
Arthritis	None, analgesics, exercise, NSAIDs, hydroxychloroquine	Low-dose systemic corticosteroids	Methotrexate	Anti-TNF	Analgesics, exercise
Renal disease	Low-dose systemic corticosteroids	High-dose systemic corticosteroids, intravenous corticosteroids	Azathioprine, IV "pulse" cyclophosphamide, mycophenolate mofetil	Cyclosporine, tacrolimus	Diet, anti-hypertensive, ACE inhibitors
Hematologic disease (cytopenias)	None	Low-dose systemic corticosteroids	Azathioprine, high-dose systemic corticosteroids, intravenous corticosteroids, rituximab	Vincristine, IV "pulse" cyclophosphamide cyclosporine, IVIG, dexamethasone, androgens, splenectomy	Transfusions GM-CSF

(continued)

TABLE 4.6 (continued)

	Minimalist treatment	May be required	Step up treatment	Occasionally used	Supportive treatment
CNS disease	Rearrange school schedule	Low-dose systemic corticosteroids	High-dose systemic corticosteroids, intravenous corticosteroids IV "pulse" cyclophosphamide	Plasmapheresis, rituximab	Anti-depressants, anti-psychotics, anti-seizure medications
Bone disease (treatment – related)	Dietary intake of appropriate calcium and vitamin D, exercise	Supplemental calcium and vitamin D	Bisphosphonate		
Anti-phospholipid antibody syndrome	Hydroxychloro-quine, avoid oral contraceptives, cardiovascular risk factors, low-dose aspirin	Anti-coagulants	Corticosteroid	Plasmapheresis, IVIG, rituximab, eculizumab	
Fatigue and malaise	Proper rest, exercise	Hydroxychloro-quine, low-dose systemic corticosteroids	Belimumab		

4.9 Neonatal Lupus Erythematosus (NLE)

The term NLE was coined to describe the syndrome in neo-nates and infants that includes skin rash, heart block, liver disease and cytopenias, and rarely other manifestations, such as bone and CNS disease. The skin and cardiac manifestations are the most frequent. These manifestations result from maternal autoantibodies, most commonly anti-Ro (SS-A) and anti-La (SS-B), which are transmitted transplacentally and attack fetal and neonatal tissues. For reasons that remain poorly understood, the mother is frequently unaffected, although she produces the autoantibodies. The presence of these autoantibodies puts her at risk, though, for the subsequent development of an autoimmune disease associ-ated with anti-Ro and anti-La antibodies, typically either SLE or Sjögren Syndrome. Pregnant women with either of these diseases who have anti-Ro and anti-La antibodies are at risk to deliver affected infants, albeit a low risk, less than 5 % [14].

Approximately 50 % of affected infants develop an annu-lar erythematous macular skin rash several weeks after birth (Fig. 4.4) or after being placed under phototherapy lights. The

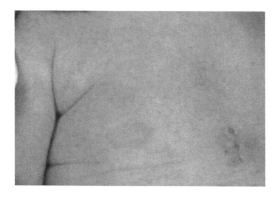

FIGURE 4.4 Scaly annular erythema lesions on the trunk of a baby with NLE: approximately 50 % of affected infants develop an annu-lar erythematous macular skin rash several weeks after birth or after being placed under phototherapy lights

rash generally disappears by 6 months of life (concurrent with the disappearance of maternal antibodies from the infant) without complication. Occasionally, at birth there is a raccoon-like periorbital or malar rash that is more deeply erythematous and scaly (Fig. 4.5). This may heal with residual scarring, atrophy, hyperpigmentation, and telangiectasia.

Congenital heart block (CHB) is the second most common manifestation of NLE. It occurs in isolation in about 50 % of cases and affects boys more than girls. CHB coexists with cutaneous NLE in about 10 % of cases. NLE is the most common cause of "idiopathic" CHB in children, and results for maternal anti-Ro and anti-La antibodies should be obtained in all cases of CHB. The block is at the level of the AV node and is an irreversible third-degree block. While it may be detected in the last part of the second trimester, often it is not recognized until the mother is in labor and the bradycardia is mistaken for fetal distress. Rarely, the bradycardia is so severe that intrauterine congestive heart failure with hydrops fetalis develops. With time, virtually all affected infants will require a pacemaker. Rarely, endocardial fibroelastosis may develop in association with NLE. Prenatal treatment with fluorinated corticosteroids may result in improved outcomes [15]. Beta-adrenergic stimulants are occasionally tried when the fetal heart rate is in the range of 50 beats per minute or below. Some experts advocate the use of IVIG. Maternal administration of hydroxychloroquine may be effective in primary prevention [16].

4.10   Drug Induced Lupus

Multiple agents have been associated with drug-induced lupus. Clinically this is usually milder than SLE, usually with less than four criteria (frequently arthritis and/or polyserositis), and will remit several months after the inciting agent is stopped. It typically occurs more in elderly Caucasians and has almost an equal frequency between males and females. The most common agent responsible for pediatric drug

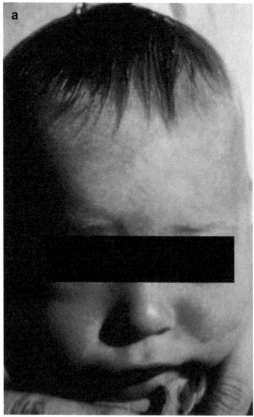

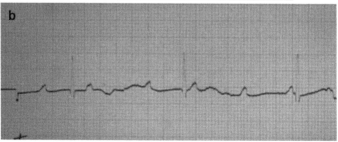

FIGURE 4.5 (**a**) Raccoon-like periorbital or malar rash that is more deeply erythematous and scaly. (**b**) ECG changes in NLE, showing AV heart block

induced lupus is minocycline, but it is also associated with chlorpromazine, hydralazine, isoniazid, and many anti-convulsant medications, among others. Serologically anti-histone antibodies are characteristic with the absence of anti-dsDNA and anti-Sm antibodies, and the complement levels are typically normal. Removal of the offending agent should lead to resolution of symptoms, but short-term ther-apy with NSAIDs, hydroxychloroquine or low-dose cortico-steroids may be warranted for symptomatic relief.

References

1. Pineles D, Valente A, Warren B, et al. Worldwide incidence and prevalence of pediatric onset systemic lupus erythematosus. Lupus. 2011;20:1187–92.
2. Benseler S, Silverman ED. Systemic lupus erythematosus. Pediatr Clin N Am. 2005;52:443–67.
3. Tan EM, Cohen AS, Fries JF, et al. The 1982 revised criteria for the classification of systemic lupus erythematosus. Arthritis Rheum. 1982;25:1271–7.
4. Hochberg MC. Updating the American College of Rheumatology revised criteria for the classification of systemic lupus erythema-tosus. Arthritis Rheum. 1997;40:1725.
5. Ferraz MB, Goldenberg J, Hilario MO, et al. Evaluation of the 1982 ARA lupus criteria data set in pediatric patients. Committees of Pediatric Rheumatology of the Brazilian Society of Pediatrics and the Brazilian Society of Rheumatology. Clin Exp Rheumatol. 1994;12:83–7.
6. Petri M, Orbai AM, Alarcón GS, et al. Derivation and validation of the Systemic Lupus International Collaborating Clinics clas-sification criteria for systemic lupus erythematosus. Arthritis Rheum. 2012;64:2677–86.
7. The American College of Rheumatology nomenclature and case definitions for neuropsychiatric lupus syndromes. Arthritis Rheum. 1999;42:599–608.
8. Muscal E, Brey RL. Neurologic manifestations of systemic lupus erythematosus in children and adults. Neurol Clin. 2010;28:61–73.
9. Hagelberg S, Lee Y, Bargman J, et al. Longterm followup of childhood lupus nephritis. J Rheumatol. 2002;29:2635–42.

10. Weening JJ, D'Agati VD, Schwartz MM, et al. The classification of glomerulonephritis in systemic lupus erythematosus revisited. J Am Soc Nephrol. 2004;15:241–50.
11. Wilson WA, Gharavi AE, Koike T, et al. International consensus statement on preliminary classification criteria for definite antiphospholipid syndrome: report of an international workshop. Arthritis Rheum. 1999;42:1309–11.
12. Avcin T. Antiphospholipid syndrome in children. Curr Opin Rheumatol. 2008;20:595–600.
13. Mina R, von Scheven E, Ardoin SP, et al. Consensus treatment plans for induction therapy of newly diagnosed proliferative lupus nephritis in juvenile systemic lupus erythematosus. Arthritis Care Res (Hoboken). 2012;64:375–83.
14. Buyon JP, Clancy RM. Neonatal lupus: basic research and clinical perspectives. Rheum Dis Clin N Am. 2005;31:299–313.
15. Saleeb S, Copel J, Friedman D, et al. Comparison of treatment with fluorinated glucocorticoids to the natural history of autoantibody-associated congenital heart block: retrospective review of the research registry for neonatal lupus. Arthritis Rheum. 1999;41:2335–45.
16. Saxena A, Izmirly PM, Mendez B, et al. Prevention and treatment in utero of autoimmune-associated congenital heart block. Cardiol Rev. 2014;22:263–7.

Chapter 5
Juvenile Dermatomyositis

5.1 Introduction

Juvenile dermatomyositis (JDM) is the most common idiopathic inflammatory myositis in children. Its presentation is unique, with characteristic skin and muscle pathology. JDM is clinically distinct from adult dermatomyositis, because it is a systemic vasculopathy, is almost never associated with malignancy, overlaps with other childhood inflammatory connective tissue diseases, and generally remits after several years.

5.2 Definition

JDM is a vasculopathy that primarily involves skin and muscle. Patients with JDM typically fulfil the criteria of Bohan and Peter or that of Targoff et al. (Table 5.1) [1–3]. Currently, many rheumatologists do not obtain EMGs or muscle biopsies unless the diagnosis is in doubt. Many will obtain a muscle MRI to look for muscle edema which is seen on STIR or T2-weighted with fat suppression images. This is very sensitive but not entirely specific as changes of edema may also be seen early in the course of muscular dystrophies, in which case a biopsy of affected muscle is essential.

R.M. Laxer et al., *Pediatric Rheumatology in Clinical Practice*,   91
DOI 10.1007/978-3-319-13099-6_5,
© Springer-Verlag London 2016

TABLE 5.1 Criteria to establish a diagnosis of JDM and JPM

No.	Criteria	Bohan and Peter criteria	Targoff et al. criteria
1.	Typical skin rash (heliotrope eyelid rash, Gottron sign, papules over extensor surfaces)	Definite JDM: criterion 1 plus 3 out of the 4 others (nos. 2–5)	Definite JDM: criteria 1 plus 3 out of the other 5 (nos. 2–6)
2.	Symmetrical proximal muscle weakness	Probable JDM: criterion 1 plus 2 out of the 4 others (nos. 2–5)	Probable JDM: criterion 1 plus 2 out of the other 5 (nos. 2–6)
3.	Elevation of serum skeletal muscle enzymes (CK, LDH, ALT, AST, aldolase)		
4.	Specific EMG changes (polyphasic decreased amplitude/duration, positive sharp waves), spontaneous insertional, high frequency, repetitive discharges	For juvenile polymyositis, criterion 1 is excluded and criteria as from JDM otherwise	This classification adds myositis-specific antibodies as a separate criterion of equal weight
5.	Specific muscle biopsy abnormalities (perifascicular degeneration, regeneration, necrosis, phagocytosis, interstitial mononuclear cell infiltrate)		Positive MRI findings may be substituted for criterion 4 or 5
6.	Myositis-specific antibodies (anti-synthetase, Mi-2, SRP, MDA-5)		

Abbreviations: *JDM* juvenile dermatomyositis, *JPM* juvenile polymyositis, *CK* creatine kinase, *LDH* lactate dehydrogenase, *ALT* alanine aminotransferase, *AST* aspartate aminotransferase, *EMG* electromyogram, *SRP* signal recognition particle, *MDA* melanoma differentiation-associated

5.3 Epidemiology

Girls are twice as likely to get JDM as boys. The peak age of onset is between 4 and 10 years. Incidence estimates have ranged from 1.9 per million individuals aged 16 and below in the UK to 3.2/million/year in children aged 2–17 in the US [4, 5].

5.4 Etiology and Pathogenesis

A number of factors have been implicated in the etiology of JDM. They include infectious, maternal microchimerism, genetic (HLA and non-HLA associated) and environmental exposures. Many of these are statistically associated but none have been proven to be clearly causative.

The disease is associated with an immune complex vasculopathy primarily involving small blood vessels in the muscle and skin. A type 1 interferon response and upregulation of MHC Class 1 molecules appear to be central to the pathogenesis of JDM. The terminal complement proteins (C5-C9) form a membrane attack complex in blood vessels.

5.5 Clinical Manifestations

There are several different presentations, outlined below.

5.5.1 Classical JDM

Constitutional features that include fatigue, malaise and fever are common early in the disease. Proximal muscle involvement leads to a fairly characteristic clinical presentation. Shoulder girdle involvement leads to an inability to raise the arms over the head and difficulty with brushing hair and reaching above the head. Weakness of the trunk muscles results in difficulty standing up straight, excessive lordosis

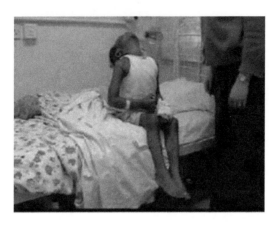

FIGURE 5.1   Proximal muscle weakness, as shown by weak neck flexors

and difficulty turning and getting in and out of bed. Weakness of the neck flexors (Fig. 5.1) results in an inability to hold the neck up when sitting. Weakness of the pelvic girdle results in difficulty negotiating stairs and a waddling gait. In severe cases, there is significant muscle edema with tenderness. Muscle tenderness distinguishes myositis from myopathy due to metabolic and genetic causes. Joint contractures due to discomfort and muscle shortening can be the presenting feature. Other manifestations of severe weakness include dysphagia with risk of aspiration and a nasal tone to the voice. Arthritis is commonly found.

The heliotrope rash around the eyes is characteristic of JDM (Fig. 5.2a). Gottron papules, scaly erythematous papules predominantly distributed over the metacarpophalangeal (MCP) and proximal interphalangeal (PIP) joints as well as over other extensor surfaces such as the knees and elbows, are another characteristic skin finding (Fig. 5.2b). Occasionally a facial rash is seen, similar to the malar rash of lupus except it does affect the nasolabial folds. Nailfold capillary changes can often be seen with the naked eye and include red and hypertrophic cuticles. A closer look with a magnified view often reveals dilated capillaries and areas of dropout. Other

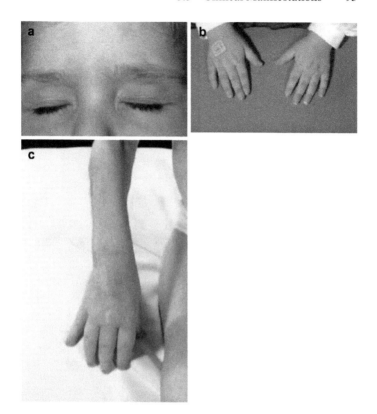

FIGURE 5.2 Skin findings in JDM. (**a**) Heliotrope rash. (**b**) Gottron papules. (**c**) Soft tissue edema

skin findings include a rash in the v-shaped area of the neck that may be an area of photosensitivity as well as a rash over the shawl area. "Mechanic's hands" may be seen in specific JDM subsets. A late finding in patients with more severe disease is lipodystrophy, which can be localized or generalized. Patients often also have hyperinsulinism, hypertriglyceridemia and acanthosis nigricans, features of the "metabolic syndrome". Edema of the affected skin and underlying tissues is another feature (Fig. 5.2c). Calcinosis is usually a late manifestation, usually 1–2 years after onset (Fig. 5.3). Risk factors

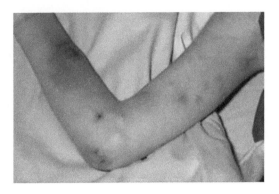

FIGURE 5.3   Calcinosis in JDM

for its development are delay in treatment and under-treatment.

Dysphonia often manifests as a higher pitch (bird-like) voice. Involvement of the chest muscles can compromise breathing and artificial ventilation is required in the severest cases. Abdominal pain, difficulty in swallowing and reflux are due to GI dysmotility. More rarely, the myocardium can be affected.

5.5.2   Amyopathic Dermatomyositis

JDM can involve skin alone (thus, sine myositis, amyopathic oy hypomyopathic dermatomyositis), although often detailed testing of muscle strength, measurement of serum levels of muscle enzymes and MRI reveals a proportion of these to have subtle muscle involvement.

5.5.3   JDM with Vasculopathy

Ulcerative disease is the most severe form of JDM. It is associated with classic nailfold capillary changes, showing damaged and blocked small arteries, veins and capillaries. The typical histological appearances are occluded and damaged

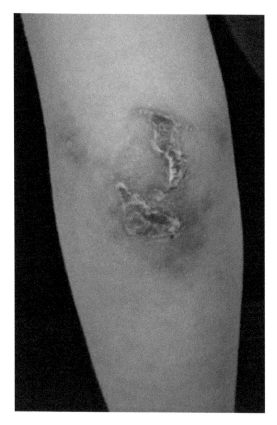

FIGURE 5.4 Skin ulcers in JDM

blood vessels, as well as inflammation. Cutaneous ulcers may occur (Fig. 5.4), usually in the axillary folds and inner canthi of the eyes. Inflammation and blockage of the vasa vasorum of the gastrointestinal (GI) tract can lead to multiple perforations of the whole GI tract (usually the stomach and small intestine) and pneumatosis intestinalis. Pulmonary vasculitis leads to spontaneous pneumothorax, and rarely, pulmonary interstitial disease can occur. Abdominal pain or sudden respiratory distress in the presence of skin ulceration, or other signs of vasculopathy, should be evaluated and treated as an emergency. This group of patients has a relapsing and chronic course with a high risk of developing calcinosis. Myocarditis is rarely seen. Central nervous system involvement may present with hallucinations or seizures, and MRI of the brain shows characteristic edematous lesions.

5.5.4   JDM with Associated Rheumatic Disease

JDM can present with features of arthritis, SLE, or systemic sclerosis (see Chap. 7). This is now known as juvenile connective tissue myositis.

5.5.5   Polymyositis

Polymyositis (PM) is much less common than JDM and many pursue more intensive evaluation given the differential diagnosis (Table 5.2), including muscle biopsy. Polymyositis tends to be more chronic and resistant to therapy than JDM.

5.6   Laboratory Features

The serum levels of muscle enzymes are almost invariably elevated. The creatine kinase (CK) is usually 5–20 times normal. Very high levels suggest rhabdomyolysis or muscular dystrophy. The other enzymes, alanine aminotransferase (ALT), aspartate aminotransferase (AST), lactic dehydrogenase (LDH) and aldolase, should be measured since some patients will have only one or two elevated enzymes. Enzymes are useful for diagnosis in the early stages of the disease, but CK often returns to normal as the muscle bulk shrinks due to damage and atrophy. Therefore CK cannot be relied upon to indicate cessation of inflammation. Muscle biopsies are indicated only if the diagnosis is in question, especially if there is no rash or an atypical rash (Table 5.2). It is best to have an ultrasound or MRI directed biopsy. EMGs are rarely indicated.

TABLE 5.2 Differential diagnosis for juvenile dermatomyositis/polymyositis

Conditions	Examples
Conditions that may be associated with rashes:	
Other idiopathic inflammatory myositis	Focal myositis, eosinophilic myositis, sarcoidosis-associated myositis
Other connective tissue disorders	Systemic lupus erythematosus, mixed connective tissue disease, scleroderma, other overlap syndromes
Infection-related myositis	Staphylococcus, toxoplasmosis, influenza, coxsackie, trichinosis
Conditions that are not associated with rashes:	
Neuromuscular disorders	
Muscular dystrophies	
Metabolic and enzyme disorders	Mitochondrial cytopathies, glycogen storage diseases
Endocrinopathies	Thyroid and parathyroid disease, Cushing disease, Addison disease
Myasthenia gravis	
Periodic paralysis	
Myotonia congenita	

In JDM with vasculopathy, the acute phase markers such as ESR and CRP, as well as other non-specific markers of inflammation are often raised. Serum levels of factor-VIII related antigen reflect endothelial damage and are often elevated in early disease.

In approximately 50 % cases of JDM, there is a positive ANA. Recently myositis-specific autoantibodies (MSA) and myositis-associated autoantibodies (MAA) have been reported to occur in a significant number of patients. The MSAs define disease subsets which may predict response to

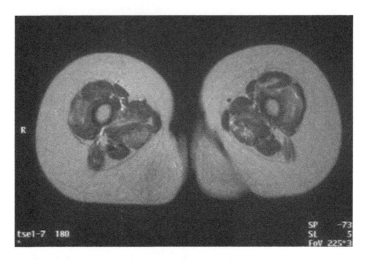

FIGURE 5.5 MRI of the thigh muscle, T2 weighted image, showing patchy inflammation of muscle groups and fasciitis

treatment [6]. MAAs are usually seen in patients with overlap syndromes.

5.7   MRI

STIR imaging or T2 weighted imaging with fat suppression can document edema within specific muscle groups and may eventually become a criterion upon which to make a diagnosis of JDM, replacing EMG (Fig. 5.5). It may also be helpful late in disease differentiating whether weakness is from fat replacement, scarring and fibrosis or ongoing inflammation.

5.8   Making the Diagnosis

The differential diagnoses are listed in Table 5.2. The Bohan and Peter diagnostic criteria and the more recent Targoff et al. criteria are listed in Table 5.1.

Most clinicians will diagnose JDM if there are at least three of the following features:

- Characteristic skin rashes
- Symmetrical proximal muscle weakness
- Elevation of skeletal muscle enzymes
- MRI evidence of muscle inflammation on T2 echo with fat suppression

5.9 Assessment of Disease Activity

A number of tools are now available to document disease activity, function and track response to treatment [7]. The Childhood Myositis Assessment Scale (CMAS) should be performed on all patients at diagnosis and on follow-up visits to help determine treatment response. There are also some specific measures of cutaneous activity. These will all be important not only for patient care but also to allow future therapeutic trials to be assessed and compared. A minimal dataset has recently been proposed to assess and follow patients allowing for better clinical trial data and comparison between different series [8].

5.10 Treatment

As with all chronic diseases, supportive care is a cornerstone of management, including skin care and physical rehabilitation. Special attention must be paid to the psychosocial aspects of a potentially debilitating disease and also the impact of medication side-effects.

Oral corticosteroid is the standard method of achieving disease control. Long-term high-dose corticosteroid is not advisable, because of growth retardation, osteoporosis, and multiple additional side effects. The Childhood Arthritis and Rheumatology Research Alliance (CARRA) has proposed three treatment regimens for initial management that will eventually be evaluated in a comparative effectiveness study (Table 5.3) [9, 10]. These include prednisone (oral ± IV),

TABLE 5.3 CARRA clinical treatment protocols for the treatment of juvenile dermatomyositis (From Huber et al. [10]) with permission from Wiley

Protocol A	Protocol B	Protocol C
Intravenous methylprednisolone	Intravenous methlyprednisolone	
30 mg/kg/day (max 1 g) × 3	30 mg/kg/day (max 1 g) × 3	
May continue 1×/week (optional)	May continue 1×/week (optional)	
Methotrexate (subcutaneous unless only oral possible)	Methotrexate (subcutaneous unless only oral possible)	Methotrexate (subcutaneous unless only oral possible)
Lesser of 15 mg/m^2 or 1 mg/kg (maximum 40 mg) once weekly	Lesser of 15 mg/m^2 or 1 mg/kg (maximum 40 mg) once weekly	Lesser of 15 mg/m^2 or 1 mg/kg (maximum 40 mg) once weekly
Prednisone	Prednisone	Prednisone
2 mg/kg/day (max 60 mg) once daily × 4 weeks, then decrease by 20 %[a]	2 mg/kg/day (max 60 mg) once daily × 4 weeks, then decrease by 20 %[a]	2 mg/kg/day (max 60 mg) divided twice daily × 4 weeks, then consolidate to once daily[a]
	Intravenous Immunoglobulin	
	2 g/kg (max 70 g), q 2 weeks × 3, then monthly	
	Optional intravenous methylprednisolone × 1 with each dose	

Summary of medication therapy in three consensus protocols for the initial treatment of moderately severe juvenile dermatomyositis (JDM)
[a]Subsequent weaning of prednisone to be determined by treating physician

methotrexate and intravenous immunoglobulin (IVIG). If gastrointestinal disease is a prominent feature, consideration should be given to administering all medications parenterally as absorption can be impaired. For patients who have not responded adequately or are steroid-dependent, treatment with cyclosporine, mycophenolate mofetil or rituximab may be considered.

Severe skin disease can be a problem in spite of systemic therapy. Hydroxychloroquine or quinacrine (mepracrine) have been advocated, but the response is not dramatic. Some success has been achieved with topical tacrolimus and intra-venous immunoglobulins may help.

In the presence of profound myositis or GI or pulmonary vasculopathy, IV cyclophosphamide has been used in addition to IV methylprednisolone. IVIG has a dramatic effect on some patients.

Physiotherapy is critical in the management of JDM, as soon as the inflammation is under control, to preserve range of motion and regain strength. Physiotherapist guided exercise to lengthen and strengthen muscles does not increase muscle inflammation. Thus, patients are likely to achieve better function if appropriate physiotherapy is instituted and the patient is not put to bed rest alone. Patients with swallowing difficulty should be nasogatric tube fed until they can safely swallow as documented by cine-esophagogram.

5.11   Course and Outcome

Classical JDM usually has a monocyclic course. A chronic or polycyclic course has been associated with more severe disease at onset, a documented infection within 6 months of onset and the presence of myositis-specific or myositis-associated antibodies [11]. Relapsing JDM is usually associated with vasculopathy. Relapse of classical JDM can occur many years after remission and after the patient has come off treatment. Mortality in a large series of patients with juvenile myositis was 4.2 % with a standardized mortality ratio of 14.4.

Juvenile connective tissue myositis and PM were associated with higher mortality rates as was severe disease at onset, older age at diagnosis, delay to diagnosis and weight loss [12].

If there is severe muscle damage during the disease, function and strength will be compromised. The CK can rise as a result of daily sporting activities, rather than as a result of myositis. In such a situation, MRI of proximal muscle groups can help assess the reason for the raised CK and avoid unnecessary steroid therapy.

Calcinosis of the soft tissue usually indicates severe disease and is associated with significant muscle damage. This can regress once the disease is in remission but may take years. Surgical removal of lumps can be helpful to prevent skin ulcerations at bony prominences. There is no evidence for specific medical treatment to reduce the calcinosis, but it is worth noting that it can be prevented by early diagnosis and aggressive induction of remission.

References

1. Bohan A, Peter JB. Polymyositis and dermatomyositis (first of two parts). N Engl J Med. 1975;292:344–7.
2. Bohan A, Peter JB. Polymyositis and dermatomyositis (second of two parts). N Engl J Med. 1975;292:403–7.
3. Targoff IN, Miller FW, Medsger Jr TA, Oddis CV. Classification criteria for the idiopathic inflammatory myopathies. Curr Opin Rheumatol. 1997;9:527–35.
4. Symmons DP, Sills JA, Davis SM. The incidence of juvenile dermatomyositis: results from a nation-wide study. Br J Rheumatol. 1995;34:732–6.
5. Mendez EP, Lipton R, Ramsey-Goldman R, et al. US incidence of juvenile dermatomyositis, 1995–1998: results from the National Institute of Arthritis and Musculoskeletal and Skin Diseases Registry. Arthritis Rheum. 2003;49:300–5.
6. Rider LG, Shah M, Mamyrova G, et al. The myositis autoantibody phenotypes of the juvenile idiopathic inflammatory myopathies. Medicine (Baltimore). 2013;92:223–43.

7. Rider LG, Werth VP, Huber AM, et al. Measures of adult and juvenile dermatomyositis, polymyositis, and inclusion body myositis: physician and patient/parent global activity, Manual Muscle Testing (MMT), Health Assessment Questionnaire (HAQ)/ Childhood Health Assessment Questionnaire (C-HAQ), Childhood Myositis Assessment Scale (CMAS), Myositis Disease Activity Assessment Tool (MDAAT), Disease Activity Score (DAS), Short Form 36 (SF-36), Child Health Questionnaire (CHQ), physician global damage, Myositis Damage Index (MDI), Quantitative Muscle Testing (QMT), Myositis Functional Index-2 (FI-2), Myositis Activities Profile (MAP), Inclusion Body Myositis Functional Rating Scale (IBMFRS), Cutaneous Dermatomyositis Disease Area and Severity Index (CDASI), Cutaneous Assessment Tool (CAT), Dermatomyositis Skin Severity Index (DSSI), Skindex, and Dermatology Life Quality Index (DLQI). Arthritis Care Res (Hoboken). 2011;63 Suppl 11:S118–57.

8. McCann LJ, Arnold K, Pilkington CA, et al. Developing a provisional, international minimal dataset for Juvenile Dermatomyositis: for use in clinical practice to inform research. Pediatr Rheumatol Online J. 2014;12:31.

9. Huber AM, Giannini EH, Bowyer SL, et al. Protocols for the initial treatment of moderately severe juvenile dermatomyositis: results of a Children's Arthritis and Rheumatology Research Alliance Consensus Conference. Arthritis Care Res (Hoboken). 2010;62:219–25.

10. Huber AM, Robinson AB, Reed AM, et al. Consensus treatments for moderate juvenile dermatomyositis: beyond the first two months. Results of the second Childhood Arthritis and Rheumatology Research Alliance consensus conference. Arthritis Care Res (Hoboken). 2012;64:546–53.

11. Habers GE, Huber AM, Mamyrova G, et al. Association of myositis autoantibodies, clinical features, and environmental exposures at illness onset are associated with disease course in juvenile myositis. Arthritis Rheumatol. 2016;68:761–8.

12. Huber AM, Mamyrova G, Lachenbruch PA, et al. Early illness features associated with mortality in the juvenile idiopathic inflammatory myopathies. Arthritis Care Res (Hoboken). 2014;66:732–40.

Chapter 6
Scleroderma and Related Disorders

6.1 Introduction

The scleroderma group of diseases is characterized by the presence of hard skin. One classification of the various forms of scleroderma is listed in Table 6.1. Successful treatment of these disorders continues to lag behind that of many of the other rheumatic diseases.

6.2 Etiology and Pathogenesis

Observations on the pathogenesis of scleroderma include (a) excessive production of collagen and extracellular matrix by fibroblasts, not only in the skin but also in vital organs and around blood vessels; this is often preceded by an initial inflammatory phase (especially in localized scleroderma, as seen clinically from biopsy and thermography); (b) endothelial cell injury with upregulation of vascular adhesion molecules, and (c) abnormalities of immune regulation, such as altered cytokine and chemokine balance, T-cell activation, and the presence of autoantibodies [1]. Also, interactions between environmental exposures and the individual genetic makeup are likely to be important contributors to the pathogenesis of these diseases. Maternal microchimerism may also play a role in disease pathogenesis, but this remains unclear.

R.M. Laxer et al., *Pediatric Rheumatology in Clinical Practice*, 107
DOI 10.1007/978-3-319-13099-6_6,
© Springer-Verlag London 2016

TABLE 6.1 Scleroderma and scleroderma-like disorders

Systemic sclerosis

Diffuse

Limited

Overlap syndromes

Localized scleroderma

Circumscribed/plaque morphea

Linear scleroderma

Limb

Face/head (Parry–Romberg syndrome/En coup de sabre)

Generalized

Pansclerotic

Mixed

Scleroderma-like disorders

Graft versus host disease

Eosinophilic fasciitis

Drug/toxin induced

Diabetic cheiroarthropathy

Phenylketonuria

Premature aging syndromes

6.3   Systemic Sclerosis (SSc)

6.3.1   Epidemiology

SSc constitutes much less than 1 % of most pediatric rheumatology clinic populations. In adults, the highest reported incidence is 1.9 per 100,000 with a prevalence of approximately 24 per 100,000 [2]. Females are affected much more commonly than males, and it is also more common in the Afro-American and native Indian populations. The annual incidence in children has been reported to be 0.27 cases/million population [3].

6.3.2   Clinical Manifestations

The diagnosis is usually suspected in a child who presents with Raynaud phenomenon (characteristic triphasic color change of distal body parts on exposure to cold or stress: white to blue to red) and other systemic manifestations. The differential diagnosis of Raynaud phenomenon is wide (Table 6.2). Raynaud phenomenon is such an important feature of SSc that its absence should always lead one to question the diagnosis of SSc. Children presenting with isolated Raynaud phenomenon alone may go on to develop SSc. Hints that the Raynaud phenomenon is likely to evolve to another illness include asymmetry, abnormal nailfold vasculature (Fig. 6.1) and the presence of a positive antinuclear antibody (ANA).

The earliest skin manifestation of SSc is non-pitting inflammatory edema of the hands, which results in restricted movement. With time, this evolves to skin thickening and tightness with an inability to pinch and lift the skin. Clinical methods to quantify skin thickening (modified Rodnan skin score) have been validated in adults but not in children. The skin may appear shiny. Progressive thickening and tightness of the skin result in joint contractures and tight skin on the face resulting in an inability to fully open the mouth (Fig. 6.2). In addition, there is a progressive loss of hair follicles. Other skin manifestations include calcinosis (Fig. 6.3), telangiectasia, and areas of skin breakdown over pressure points. If digital blood flow is particularly compromised, digital pitting, ulceration and even gangrenous changes may develop. Areas of hyperpigmentation and hypopigmentation can result in a "salt and pepper" appearance. The distribution of thickening differs in the two major types of SSc (diffuse and limited). Involvement proximal to the wrist and

TABLE 6.2 Differential Diagnosis of Raynaud phenomenon

Primary

Secondary

  Connective tissue disease

    Scleroderma

    Mixed connective tissue disease

    Systemic lupus erythematosus

    Dermatomyositis

    Overlap syndromes

  Mechanical obstruction

    Thoracic outlet syndrome

    Cervical rib

  Drug/toxin induced

  Cryoglobulinemia

  Polycythemia

Vibratory worker

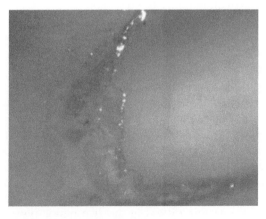

FIGURE 6.1 Abnormal nailfold capillary microscopy

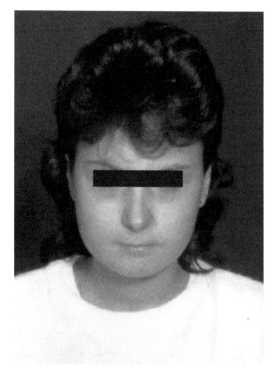

FIGURE 6.2 Tight skin on the face of a 14-year-old girl with diffuse systemic sclerosis

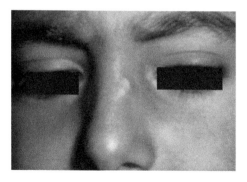

FIGURE 6.3 Calcinosis over the nasal bridge in an 8-year-old boy with systemic sclerosis

ankles, and involvement of the trunk, is more characteristic of diffuse disease which has a higher rate of internal organ involvement and earlier clinical manifestations of internal organ dysfunction. Limited SSc (formerly known as CREST syndrome) progresses much more slowly, but there is a greater risk of the late development of pulmonary hypertension.

Musculoskeletal involvement is common. Fibrosis of the joint capsule and thickening of the synovium lead to joint contractures, a problem exacerbated by the thickened and tight skin around the joint. The joints may be tender but are not usually swollen. A subclinical myopathy, with minimal weakness and mild elevation of serum levels of muscle enzymes, is common. More significant muscle involvement can occasionally occur, especially when there is an overlap with the myositis syndromes. Another characteristic feature, tendon friction rubs, can be felt and heard over the wrists and ankles; their presence seems to predict a poor outcome overall.

Gastrointestinal involvement is a major cause of morbidity (Table 6.3). Dysphagia results from both oral dryness and poor esophageal peristalsis secondary to esophageal fibrosis. Dysfunction of the lower esophageal sphincter results in acid reflux and the potential for the development of reflux esophagitis. Dysmotility of the small intestine may lead to stasis, bacterial overgrowth and malabsorption with diarrhea. Finally, severe constipation and megacolon occasionally occur.

Renal disease, formerly the major cause of mortality, is now more manageable with the advent of angiotensin converting enzyme inhibitors. Renal vasculopathy may lead to the development of "scleroderma kidney," which usually presents with hypertension and microangiopathy. This potentially catastrophic complication may be precipitated by high-dose corticosteroids. The hypertension may be preceded by proteinuria. Glomerular disease is rare.

The major current cause of mortality results from pulmonary involvement, which can take several forms (Table 6.4). Interstitial lung disease begins as an inflammatory alveolitis

TABLE 6.3 Gastrointestinal manifestations of scleroderma

Reduced oral aperture

Oral sicca

Dysphagia

Esophageal reflux (may result in esophagitis and persistent ulceration) with heartburn

Nocturnal aspiration

Cough with swallowing

Delayed gastric emptying

Gastric antral vascular ectasia (watermelon stomach)

Bacterial overgrowth with malabsorption

Megacolon with constipation

Diarrhea

Incontinence

TABLE 6.4 Pleuropulmonary manifestations of systemic sclerosis

Pleural effusion

Inflammatory alveolitis

Interstitial fibrosis

Pulmonary hypertension

Recurrent aspiration pneumonia

which evolves to interstitial fibrosis. It is critical to discover the lung disease in its early stage when it may still be responsive to treatment. The second most common form of pulmonary disease is pulmonary hypertension, which can occur in isolation as part of the vasculopathy of scleroderma, or secondary to the interstitial lung disease. Symptoms include dyspnea and hypoxemia. This can usually be detected by echocardiography. Recurrent nocturnal aspiration from lower esophageal dysfunction may also lead to chronic lung disease. Finally, pleuritis with or without pleural effusion may also occur. Early symptoms of pulmonary involvement include dry cough, followed by progressive dyspnea on exertion. On examination, dry rales may be heard as the disease progresses and may be associated with reduced chest expansion.

The heart is also commonly affected. Pericarditis (usually asymptomatic) with small pericardial effusions is very common. Involvement of the cardiac microvasculature leads to tiny areas of microinfarcton, which can eventually result in a cardiomyopathy. Involvement of the conducting system by fibrosis can result in bundle branch block or other arrhythmias.

Other systemic involvement includes periodontal ligaments with dental loosening, bony resorption, rare neuropathies (e.g., trigeminal), sicca syndrome and thyroid involvement.

6.3.3   Investigations

Laboratory features can be divided into those that are non-specific and reflect the presence and degree of organ involvement, and those that are more specific to the different forms of scleroderma (Table 6.5). Laboratory signs of systemic inflammation are generally absent, except early in the disease course where the erythrocyte sedimentation rate (ESR) and other markers of acute inflammation may be elevated. Anemia may result from poor diet, malabsorption or chronic disease. Signs of endothelial activation are reflected in a raised von Willebrand factor antigen. Mild elevations of serum levels of muscle enzymes accompany the scleroderma myopathy and these are significantly raised in overlap syndromes (see Chap. 7). It is important to monitor pulmonary function tests. Early disease is reflected in a reduced diffusing capacity of carbon monoxide (DLCO), while progressive fibrosis is shown by a reduced residual volume and forced vital capacity and FEV1. High resolution, thin-section CT scan of the lungs is critically important in the evaluation of patients. Early alveolitis is shown by the presence of ground-glass appearance, primarily in the lung bases, before the development of fibrosis. The presence of pulmonary hypertension may be sought by cardiac echocardiography, although

TABLE 6.5 Suggested investigations for systemic sclerosis

System/organ	Investigations
Immune	ANA, RF, anti-Scl 70, anti-centromere
Renal	Urinalysis for proteinuria
Cardiac	ECG (rhythm), echocardiogram (effusion, pulmonary hypertension)
Pulmonary	Pulmonary function tests with diffusing capacity carbon monoxide (DLCO), chest radiograph, high resolution CT scan
Gastrointestinal	Swallowing study (reflux, strictures)

at intermediate levels of pulmonary hypertension a right side cardiac catheterization may be required. An electrocardiogram should be done to detect the presence of arrhythmias and right ventricular hypertrophy. Renal abnormalities are uncommon until proteinuria indicates the onset of "scleroderma kidney" with renovascular hypertension and microangiopathic hemolytic anemia and thrombocytopenia.

Serologic abnormalities are common and help classify patients. Nonspecific antinuclear antibodies, usually with a speckled or nucleolar pattern, are seen in 80–90 % of patients, and rheumatoid factor positivity in a minority of patients. The specificity of the ANA is important. The presence of anti Scl-70 (antitopoisomerase I) correlates with diffuse SSc, and anticentromere antibodies with limited SSc. Other autoantibodies may occur; anti-PM-Scl and anti-U1-RNP are seen in overlap syndromes with myositis as a prominent feature. More specific autoantibodies can be looked for to help determine risk of specific organ involvement but are generally available only on a research basis.

6.3.4 Course and Outcome

The course of SSc is usually characterized by skin tightening with eventual softening over time. Unfortunately, organ dysfunction is progressive over several years, at which point there is either stabilization or progressive dysfunction. The outcome is determined by the rate of progression of internal organ manifestations in the first few years after presentation. In general, the outcome is better than in adult SSc [4]. Severe early skin thickening is a poor prognostic indicator in adults with SSc.

6.3.5   Treatment

Treating patients with scleroderma continues to be very frustrating for patients and practitioners. Most important have been the advances in treating end-organ manifestations. Treatment should be considered in terms of (1) the disease process itself, (2) end organ manifestations, and (3) general supportive measures. A series of evidence-based recommendations has been published recently [5].

To date, no treatment has been proven definitively to alter the course of SSc. Immunomodulatory agents, which may be effective include methotrexate, mycophenolate mofetil, cyclophosphamide, rituximab, tocilizumab and antithymocyte globulin. Further studies are required and are ongoing. Autologous stem cell transplantation may be considered in patients with progressive but potentially reversible pulmonary or cardiac disease.

The morbidity of SSc has been dramatically altered due to the availability of agents to treat the organ-specific disease manifestations. Table 6.6 lists the treatment options for the various end-organ manifestations.

6.3.6   Making the Diagnosis

New classification criteria for systemic sclerosis were published that have a better sensitivity and specificity than those originally published and they may be applied to children as

TABLE 6.6 Treatment of end-organ manifestations of systemic sclerosis

Manifestation	Supportive measure	Pharmacologic treatment
Raynaud phenomenon	Keep warm	Peripheral vasodilators (e.g., calcium channel blockers [nifedipine, nocardipine], losartan, topical nitroglycerine); May also consider phosphodiesterase inhibitors such as sildenafil, IV prostaglandins and endothelin-1 antagonists
Skin	Keep moist, massage	Methotrexate
Reflux esophagitis/ gastrointestinal	Small meals, elevate head of bed, do not lie supine after eating	Proton pump inhibitors; consider prokinetic drugs such as octreotide, antibiotics for malabsorption syndrome
Renal disease	Appropriate diet	Angiotensin converting enzyme inhibitor
Pulmonary alveolitis		Trial of glucocorticoids and cyclophosphamide; Also consider mycophenolate mofetil, rituximab
Pulmonary hypertension		Trial of phosphodiesterase inhibitor, endothelin receptor antagonist (bosentan)

well [6] (Table 6.7). Classification criteria for childhood systemic sclerosis have also been proposed, (Table 6.8) and are currently under study [7] as is a preliminary disease severity score [8].

There are several clinical scenarios in which systemic sclerosis should be suspected even prior to the development of skin changes, as listed in Table 6.9.

TABLE 6.7 Preliminary criteria for the classification of systemic sclerosis

Category	Subitems	Weight
Skin	Skin thickening of the fingers of both hands extending proximal to the MCPs	9
	Puffy fingers	2
	Whole finger, distal to MCP	4
Fingertip lesions	Digital tip ulcers	2
	Pitting scars	3
Telangiectasia	–	2
Abnormal nailfold capillaries	–	2
PAH and/or interstitial lung disease	–	2
Raynaud phenomenon	–	3
Scleroderma-related antibodies (any of anticentromere, anti-topoisomerase-I [anti-Scl-70], anti-RNA polymerase-3)	–	3
–	Total score:	
Only the highest score from each category is used and the sum is totaled; a score of 9 or more classifies a patient as having systemic sclerosis		

From Ref. [6]
MCP Metacarpophalangeal, *PAH* pulmonary hypertension

TABLE 6.8 Preliminary classification criteria for systemic sclerosis in children [7]

Major criterion (required)

  Proximal skin sclerosis/induration of the skin

Minor criteria (at least 2 required)

  Cutaneous

    Sclerodactyly

  Peripheral vascular

    Raynaud phenomenon

    Nailfold capillary abnormalities

    Digital tip ulcers

  Gastrointestinal

    Dysphagia

    Gastroesophageal reflux

  Cardiac

    Arrhythmias

    Heart failure

  Renal

    Renal crisis

    New-onset arterial hypertension

  Respiratory

    Pulmonary fibrosis (HRCT/radiography)

    Decreased DLCO

    Pulmonary arterial hypertension

  Neurologic

    Neuropathy

    Carpal tunnel syndrome

(continued)

TABLE 6.8 (continued)

Musculoskeletal

    Tendon friction rubs

    Arthritis

    Myositis

Serologic

    Antinuclear antibodies

    SSc-selective autoantibodies (anticentromere, anti-topoisomerase I [Scl-70], antifibrillarin, anti-PM-Scl, antifibrillin or anti-RNA polymerase I or II)

The highest score was the presence of the major criterion and at least two minor criteria

DLCO diffusing capacity for carbon monoxide

HRCT high-resolution computed tomography

TABLE 6.9 When to consider systemic sclerosis

Raynaud phenomenon in the presence of a positive ANA and/or abnormal nailfold capillaries

Polyarthritis with minimal effusions

Unexplained pulmonary fibrosis

Severe gastroesophageal reflux

Unexplained pulmonary hypertension

Unexplained myopathy

Local nodular calcinosis

Hypertensive crisis

6.4   Localized Scleroderma

In children, localized forms of scleroderma (also known as morphea) are much more common than systemic ones and, while generally much milder, they can be associated with serious consequences. Like systemic disease, the unifying feature is hardening of the skin. Yet some forms considered to be part of localized scleroderma are associated with atrophy rather than hardening, and often the initial firm phase gives way to softening with atrophy. The Padua Classification includes five sub-types (Table 6.1) [9].

6.4.1 Plaque/Circumscribed Morphea

The most characteristic lesion of morphea is a plaque involving the trunk (Fig. 6.4). This usually begins as a firm, ivory colored oval lesion which may be up to several centimeters in size. Although usually asymptomatic, occasionally tingling or itching is reported. The center is usually surrounded by a reddish-lilac color ring that suggests the process is active and inflammatory. The lesion often expands over several years, but eventually softens spontaneously. As part of the healing process, atrophy with hyperpigmentation commonly develops. When there are more than four lesions in three different areas, the disorder is known as generalized morphea.

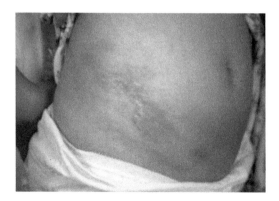

Figure 6.4 Plaque morphea lesion involving the trunk

6.4.2   Linear Scleroderma

Over 50 % of children with localized forms of scleroderma will have bands of firm sclerotic tissue in a linear distribution, classified as linear scleroderma (Fig. 6.5). The location will determine the impact and course. If the lesion crosses joints, it may result in contractures and loss of motion. It also may affect the growth, both circumferential as well as linear of the extremity and occasionally result in a withered, nonfunctional

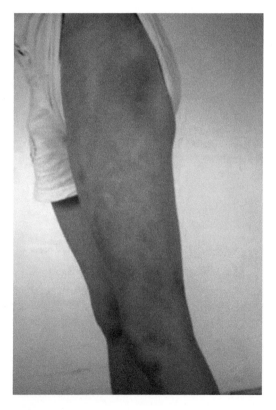

FIGURE 6.5 Linear scleroderma lesion

limb. Muscle atrophy and shortening of the extremity are not uncommon.

When linear scleroderma affects the face, the disorder is known as either scleroderma "en coup de sabre", or progressive hemifacial atrophy, also known as Parry–Romberg syndrome. En coup de sabre lesions occur on the forehead, usually in a paramedian distribution, and often extend upward into the scalp with associated localized alopecia (Fig. 6.6). Early on, the band is firm and "cuts into" the forehead and scalp with localized atrophy. It may extend through muscle and bone and result in defects in the skull vault. The band may cross the eye and "tent" the nasal ala. Uveits can occur. Deeper involvement may irritate the cerebral cortex and result in seizures. Cerebral calcifications are common, but their significance is uncertain. The lesion may extend lower to involve the lips, tongue, maxillary and mandibular bones. Patients with Parry–Romberg syndrome have significant facial deformities, which progress over time as the unaffected side continues its normal growth (Fig. 6.7). Dental abnormalities are common.

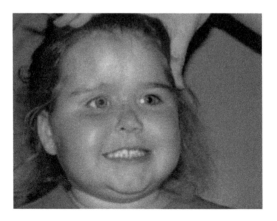

FIGURE 6.6 En coup de sabre scleroderma lesion

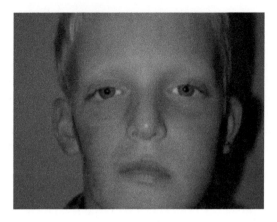

FIGURE 6.7 Parry-Romberg syndrome

6.4.3   Pansclerotic Morphea

Pansclerotic morphea is characterized by diffuse thickening which involves all extremities and the trunk but tends to spare the fingers and toes. This may result in severe contractures and restriction in chest wall movement. It is debilitating and progressive.

6.4.4   Making the Diagnosis

The diagnosis is made clinically by recognizing the characteristic lesions. When there is doubt, a skin biopsy showing thickening of the collagen bundles, usually with an inflammatory infiltrate, will confirm the diagnosis. Other cutaneous disorders which can mimic localized scleroderma include eosinophilic fasciitis, cutaneous T-cell lymphoma, lichen sclerosis et atrophicus and collagenoma. These can all be diagnosed by skin biopsy. Laboratory abnormalities can include mild elevation of the ESR or CRP, hypergammaglobulinemia, eosinophilia and a positive ANA and rheumatoid factor. However, all may be normal or negative even in active disease.

6.4.5   Treatment

For plaque morphea, topical therapy may be all that is necessary. Application of calcipotriene (with or without corticosteroids) or tacrolimus may be effective. Success has been reported with ultraviolet light therapy as well. Deep tissue massage may also be helpful. When lesions are appearing rapidly, crossing joint lines, or have the potential to result in serious cosmetic deformity and functional disability, systemic treatments should be used early to suppress the inflammatory phase, with a view to halt the progression to growth abnormalities and fibrosis. Currently, a combination of short-term corticosteroid (orally or intravenously) and longer-term methotrexate (approximately 15 mg/m^2 per week) is frequently used. While short-term efficacy of methotrexate has been shown in a placebo-controlled trial [10], a study, sponsored by the Childhood Arthritis and Rheumatology Research Alliance (CARRA) is currently underway comparing three treatment groups: methotrexate alone or with corticosteroids given either orally or intravenously [11]. In resistant disease, mycophenolate mofetil (MMF) may be considered. Surgery may be helpful for disfiguring facial lesions [12] but should only be considered when the disease had been in clinical remission for at least 1 year.

6.5   Eosinophilic Fasciitis

Described almost 40 years ago, eosinophilic fasciitis (EF) is characterized by the relatively sudden onset of extremity swelling and pain with an thickened indurated appearance like that of the skin of an orange (peau d'orange). There is a significant inflammatory infiltrate within the fascia predominated by eosinophils. Peripheral eosinophilia is not always present. There is a vigorous acute-phase response, and very high levels of serum IgG are typically seen. MRI shows the marked fascial edema and can be used to monitor response to treatment. Corticosteroids are used as first-line treatment. Steroid sparing agents such as hydroxychloroquine, methotrexate and MMF may help ease the steroid taper and can also be used for recurrent disease.

References

1. Denton CP. Systemic sclerosis: from pathogenesis to targeted therapy. Clin Exp Rheumatol. 2015;33(Suppl 92):3–7.
2. Mayes MD, Lacey Jr JV, Beebe-Dimmer J, et al. Prevalence, incidence, survival, and disease characteristics of systemic sclerosis in a large US population. Arthritis Rheum. 2003;48:2246–55.
3. Herrick AL, Ennis H, Bhushan M, Silman AJ, Baildam EM. Incidence of childhood linear scleroderma and systemic sclerosis in the UK and Ireland. Arthritis Care Res (Hoboken). 2010;62:213–8.
4. Martini G, Foeldvari I, Russo R, et al. Juvenile Scleroderma Working Group of the Pediatric Rheumatology European Society. Systemic sclerosis in childhood: clinical and immunologic features of 153 patients in an international database. Arthritis Rheum. 2006;54:3971–8.
5. Kowal-Bielecka O, Landewé R, Avouac J, et al. EULAR recommendations for the treatment of systemic sclerosis: a report from the EULAR Scleroderma Trials and Research group (EUSTAR). Ann Rheum Dis. 2009;68:620–8.
6. Distler O, Allanore Y, Furst DE, et al. 2013 classification criteria for systemic sclerosis: an American college of rheumatology/European league against rheumatism collaborative initiative. Ann Rheum Dis. 2013;72:1747–55.
7. Zulian F, Woo P, Athreya BH, et al. The Pediatric Rheumatology European Society/American College of Rheumatology/European League against Rheumatism provisional classification criteria for juvenile systemic sclerosis. Arthritis Rheum. 2007;57:203–12.
8. La Torre F, Martini G, Russo R, et al. A preliminary disease severity score for juvenile systemic sclerosis. Arthritis Rheum. 2012;64:4143–50.
9. Laxer RM, Zulian F. Localized scleroderma. Curr Opin Rheumatol. 2006;18:606–1.
10. Zulian F, Vallongo C, Patrizi A, et al. A long-term follow-up study of methotrexate in juvenile localized scleroderma (morphea). J Am Acad Dermatol. 2012;67:1151–6.

11. Li SC, Torok KS, Pope E, et al. Childhood Arthritis and Rheumatology Research Alliance (CARRA) Localized Scleroderma Workgroup. Development of consensus treatment plans for juvenile localized scleroderma: a roadmap toward comparative effectiveness studies in juvenile localized scleroderma. Arthritis Care Res (Hoboken). 2012;64:1175–85.
12. Palmero ML, Uziel Y, Laxer RM, Forrest CR, Pope E. En coup de sabre scleroderma and Parry-Romberg syndrome in adolescents: surgical options and patient-related outcomes. J Rheumatol. 2010;37:2174–9.

Chapter 7
Overlap Syndromes

7.1 Introduction

Many patients present with clinical and laboratory signs and symptoms that are compatible with several of the classic connective tissue diseases (CTD), such as juvenile idiopathic arthritis (JIA), systemic lupus erythematosus (SLE), juvenile dermatomyositis (JDM), and systemic sclerosis (SSc). These children, who have overlapping features of several CTDs, are said to have "overlap syndromes" or "undifferentiated connective tissue diseases." Patients may remain with overlapping features for many years, or their clinical picture may evolve into one of the more classic CTDs. Two overlap CTDs are better defined in terms of having diagnostic criteria and characteristic serologic features: mixed connective tissue disease (MCTD) and Sjögren syndrome (SS). In addition, two other disorders with multisystem involvement will be described: IgG4 disease, and sarcoidosis.

7.2 Mixed Connective Tissue Disease

MCTD is a disease whose manifestations include overlapping features of SLE, JIA, JDM, and SSc, with a high titer antinuclear antibody and speckled pattern on immunofluorescence, together with specific autoantibodies directed against

R.M. Laxer et al., *Pediatric Rheumatology in Clinical Practice*,   129
DOI 10.1007/978-3-319-13099-6_7,
© Springer-Verlag London 2016

the U1RNP component of the extractable nuclear antigen (ENA) complex. The presence of other specific antinuclear antibodies in significant titer should exclude the diagnosis of MCTD. MCTD, like other autoimmune diseases, has certain immunogenetic associations, suggesting that these patients are "genetically predetermined" to develop the disease. An inciting environmental agent(s) is likely critical to trigger the development of autoantibodies and disease manifestations. A variety of diagnostic criteria have been proposed for MCTD, but none have been validated in children [1].

Most commonly, early symptoms include swelling with edema of the hands (Fig. 7.1) and Raynaud phenomenon [2]. The remaining clinical manifestations are determined by which component of the "overlapping" disease is playing the most prominent role. For instance, it may be the rash and

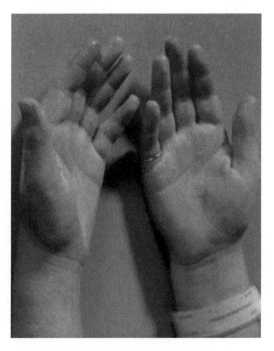

FIGURE 7.1 Picture showing "sausage fingers" seen in early MCTD

proximal muscle weakness of JDM; the esophageal distur-bance and lung disease of systemic sclerosis; the malar rash and serositis of SLE; or the polyarthritis of JIA. Severe glo-merulonephritis and thrombocytopenia are uncommon unless the MCTD evolves towards "full-blown" SLE, in which case additional autoantibodies usually develop.

7.2.1   Prevalence

MCTD is uncommon in children and represents much less than 1 % of most pediatric rheumatology clinic populations. It occurs most commonly in adolescence with a female to male ratio of approximately 5:1 [1, 2]. The usual age of onset is in the early adolescent years, but can occur in children as young as 5 years of age.

7.2.2   Natural History and Disease Course

Features at onset often include puffiness of the fingers and hands (Fig. 7.1). Raynaud phenomenon, another of the char-acteristic early features present in the majority of cases of MCTD, usually persists throughout the course, and, like with systemic sclerosis, is often severe with potential to leave digi-tal scarring. Skin signs of SLE and JDM and proximal muscle weakness are seen early in the course. The myositis may not be as severe as in JDM. Arthritis is an early feature, fre-quently persists and can lead to deformities with or without erosions. Arthritis may involve large and small joints, typi-cally in a symmetrical pattern. Tight skin may contribute to joint contractures although this is generally a later feature.

Pulmonary function abnormalities are common through-out the course, although usually asymptomatic at onset. However, with time interstitial lung disease may develop and, more rarely, pulmonary hypertension occurs. Patients must be monitored closely for the development of either of these two potentially fatal complications.

Renal disease is not common, unless the patient pursues a course more akin to SLE, in which case manifestations of glomerulonephritis and nephrotic syndrome can occur. Rarely, renal failure develops.

Other clinical manifestations include those that may occur in the diseases that contribute to the overlap. Pleuritis and pericarditis, representing contributions mainly of SLE, can occasionally occur. The classic cutaneous features of JDM, such as Gottron papules and heliotrope rash (Fig. 7.2) may be seen. The gastrointestinal manifestations associated with systemic sclerosis, such as dysphagia and reflux, often develop with time. Sicca symptoms are common. Central nervous manifestations are uncommon, unless the MCTD is dominated by features of SLE. Leukopenia and thrombocytopenia are frequent findings.

7.2.3   Diagnosis

The diagnosis is based on the combination of features of various classic autoimmune connective tissue diseases, together with the laboratory features of high titer ANA in speckled pattern and the presence of antibodies to U1RNP. No other ANA specificity should be present. It should be noted that antibodies to U1RNP may also occur, usually in lower titer, in patients with SLE and scleroderma.

7.2.4   Course and Outcome

Patients must be followed closely for evolution of organ system dysfunction and failure, especially involving the lungs and kidneys. A small number of patients may go into a full remission and not require medication [3]. However, mortality is reported in the range of 3–28 %. Deaths have resulted from infection, and are likely related to immunosuppression needed to manage the disease. Death has also been reported

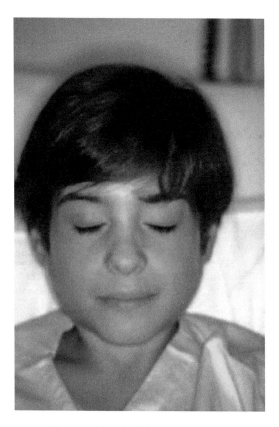

FIGURE 7.2 A 14-year-old girl with overlap syndrome who complained of joint pain as well as sudden onset of pain and swelling over the angle of both jaws: note the heliotropic discoloration over the eyelids and bilateral parotid swelling typical of Sjögren syndrome

due to severe renal disease, pulmonary hypertension and myocarditis. The course is dictated by whether the disease evolves into a lupus-like or scleroderma-like process.

Overall, approximately 75 % of patients have a favourable outcome.

7.2.5   Treatment

There is nothing specific to the treatment of MCTD other than careful attention to vital organ involvement and provision of ongoing family-centered care and psychosocial support. The reader is referred to the relevant chapters regarding treatment of the various clinical manifestations present in the patient.

7.3   Sjögren Syndrome

Sjögren syndrome (SS) is an overlap syndrome, which may occur as part of an underlying autoimmune CTD (in which case it is known as secondary SS) or in isolation, also known as primary SS [4]. Secondary SS is more common, and is seen in children most commonly with SLE, systemic sclerosis, and MCTD; it may also be seen in sarcoidosis. SS is characterized clinically by the "sicca complex" of dry eyes and dry mouth, in association with anti-Ro and anti-La antibodies (also known as anti-SS-A and anti-SS-B, respectively). Proposed classification criteria have been developed for adults [5] but may not be relevant for children. Diagnostic criteria have recently been proposed for juvenile SS (Table 7.1) [6]. In childhood, any focal sialadenitis is suggestive of the diagnosis of SS [7].

The pathology of SS is characterized by lymphocytic inflammation of exocrine glands, especially the salivary and lacrimal glands. The inciting agent that results in this attack is unknown; several authors have postulated an underlying viral etiology. Other affected glandular tissues may include the renal tubules and bile canaliculi with resultant clinical manifestations of renal tubular acidosis and primary biliary cirrhosis. The role of the autoantibodies in pathogenesis is unknown but their presence is almost universal. Upregulation of type I interferon signature genes and Th1, 2 and 17 activity are seen. Patients with SS generally have the immunogenetic phenotype HLADR3, DQw1, and DQw2.

TABLE 7.1 Proposed criteria for juvenile primary Sjögren syndrome

I. Clinical symptoms

1. Oral (dry mouth, recurrent parotitis, or enlargement of parotid glands)

2. Ocular (recurrent conjunctivitis without obvious allergic or infectious etiology, keratoconjunctivitis sicca)

3. Other mucosal involvement (recurrent vaginitis)

4. Systemic (fever of unknown origin, noninflammatory arthralgias, hypokalemic paralysis, abdominal pain)

II. Immunological abnormalities (presence of at least one of the following: anti-SS-A, anti-SS-B, high-titer ANA, RF)

III. Other laboratory abnormalities or additional investigations

1. Biochemical (elevated serum amylase)

2. Hematological (leukopenia, high ESR)

3. Immunological (polyclonal hyperimmunoglobulinemia)

4. Nephrological (renal tubular acidosis)

5. Histological proof of lymphocytic infiltration of salivary glands or other organs

6. Objective documentation of ocular dryness (Bengal red staining, Schirmer test)

7. Objective documentation of parotid gland involvement (sialography)

IV. Exclusion of all other autoimmune diseases

Presence of four more criteria required for diagnosis

From Bartunkova et al. [7]

7.3.1 Prevalence

SS is rare in childhood. Secondary SS is more common and is associated with CTDs whose incidence is increased in adolescence, SS is seen more commonly in late adolescence, but it has been reported in children as young as 5 years of age.

7.3.2   Clinical Manifestations

The clinical manifestations relate to the sicca complex primarily and to glandular inflammation. A common presenting feature in children is recurrent parotitis that is not responsive to antibiotics [8] (Fig. 7.2). With time, recurrent lymphocytic infiltration of the salivary glands will result in destruction of ductal tissue and reduced salivary flow, which will result in persistent dry mouth. On examination, there is a poor saliva pool under the tongue and the tongue blade often sticks to the tongue. Patients have difficulty initiating swallowing ("upper" dysphagia) and often have to have drink to facilitate swallowing of food and water by their bedside at night to combat a dry mouth. Dental caries become a significant problem. Ocular dryness results in photophobia with a feeling of "sand" in the eye. Vaginal dryness with dyspareunia is a major problem. Other manifestations of glandular involvement can include exocrine pancreatic dysfunction, pneumonitis and dry skin. If the SS is secondary to another CTD, symptoms and signs of that CTD may dominate. However, extraglandular signs and symptoms occur in a significant percentage of children with primary SS, including substantial fatigue, hematologic abnormalities (primarily neutropenia), cutaneous vasculitis, arthritis/arthralgias, peripheral lymphadenopathy, peripheral neuropathy and CNS involvement. Cases of acute febrile encephalitis with SS have been reported [9]. A persistent metabolic acidosis, secondary to renal tubular acidosis may rarely develop and lead to growth delay. Liver dysfunction secondary to biliary cirrhosis is occasionally seen. Neuromeyelitis optica with antibodies to aquaporin 4 may occur. B-cell lymphoma, which does occur in adults with SS, has not been reported in pediatric SS.

7.3.3   Diagnosis

SS is frequently accompanied by significant hypergammaglobulinemia, positive rheumatoid factor in high titer, positive ANA in high titer, and anti-Ro (SS-A) and anti-La

(SS-B) antibodies. Elevated levels of serum amylase are common. Importantly, antibodies to dsDNA, and cardiolipin are negative, as is ANCA, and serum complement levels are normal. Ocular dryness can be confirmed by a positive Schirmer Test (placing a strip of filter paper in the ocular sac and observing the degree of wetting over 5 min); <5 mm is considered a positive test. A Rose Bengal or lissamine green corneal stain may demonstrate corneal erosions resulting from ocular dryness. Xerostomia can be investigated by salivary scan, showing reduced salivary flow. A biopsy of minor salivary glands, demonstrating lymphocytic infiltration, may occasionally be necessary, especially when excluding other causes of parotitis. Malignancy and sarcoidosis should always be considered in the differential diagnosis.

7.3.4 Course and Outcome

Fortunately, the outcome of children with primary SS is good, although symptomatic treatment is necessary to improve their quality of life.

7.3.5 Treatment

Ocular and oral dryness are very troublesome to patients and attention to local hygiene is extremely important. Artificial tears should be used to maintain corneal hydration, and saliva substitutes have also recently become available. Careful attention must be paid to the prevention of dental caries. Oral pilocarpine may help both the oral and ocular sicca symptoms. The treatment of the systemic manifestations is based on the specific organ involvement, and usually includes NSAIDs, hydroxychloroquine, and corticosteroids. For extra glandular manifestations with life-threatening potential, treatment with corticosteroids, or more rarely, cyclophosphamide (especially for CNS disease) is necessary. Rituximab may also be considered and may be helpful for sicca symptoms as well as general improvement in global disease activity indices.

7.4   IgG4 Disease

IgG4 disease is a recently recognized disorder characterized by infiltration of various tissues and organs with inflammatory and fibrotic masses [10]. Typically, but not always, serum levels of IgG4 are raised. The diagnosis is made by the histologic features of storiform fibrosis, obliterative phlebitis and the presence of IgG4 producing plasma cells. Infiltration of salivary glands can give the appearance of Sjögren syndrome. Pancreatitis, often recurrent, was one of the very early features described in this disease. In children one of the most important presenting features is orbital pseudotumor. Other manifestations include hypertrophic pachymeningitis, retroperitoneal fibrosis and sclerosing cholangitis. Corticosteroids are a mainstay of treatment, and other options include mycophenolate mofetil and rituximab.

7.5   Sarcoidosis

Sarcoidosis is a multisystem disorder marked by the presence of non-caseating granulomatous inflammation. An early-onset form is characterized by the triad of arthritis, skin rash and uveitis; it is associated with mutations in the *NOD 2/ CARD 15* gene and is known as Blau syndrome. The adult form, (pediatric-onset adult type sarcoidosis), which occurs almost exclusively in adolescents, is discussed here [11].

Most patients present with constitutional features such as fever, anorexia, weight loss and fatigue. Typical clinical manifestations include generalized lymphadenopathy and hepatosplenomegaly. The most common cutaneous manifestation is erythema nodosum; plaques, papules and nodules are less frequent. The lungs are involved in the majority of cases with diffuse micronodular pulmonary infiltration; initially this may be sub-clinical and detected by CT scan and pulmonary function tests. The most common clinical association is cough and dyspnea. Hilar lymphadenopathy accompanies the lung disease in the majority of cases. Ocular manifestations, including conjunctivitis and anterior uveitis (usually asymptomatic) occur in about 25 % of patients. Neurosarcoid is uncommon and can present in a variety of ways including peripheral neuropathy, cerebral mass and with characteristics similar to cerebral vasculitis. Both oligoarthritis and polyarthritis may occur. Joints often have marked synovial hypertrophy with a "boggy" feeling to the joint. Bone lesions, particularly in the phalanges may occur. Cardiac involvement with arrhythmias and myocarditis may be fatal. Renal dysfunction and hypertension secondary to hypercalcemia can progress rapidly.

Most patients will have an elevated acute phase response with anemia of chronic disease, leukocytosis, thrombocytosis, raised ESR and CRP and hypergammaglobulinemia. Many patients will have liver enzyme abnormalities and are particularly sensitive to medications with liver adverse effects. Chest x-ray can show hilar lymphadenopathy and pulmonary infiltrates; sometimes a CT scan is required to demonstrate these changes. Hypercalciuria is common and hypercalcemia may be seen as well. Angiotensin-converting enzyme levels are not specific enough to confirm a diagnosis, especially in African Americans where normal may be higher than in Caucasians. The finding of non-caseating granulomata on biopsy is extremely helpful in confirming the diagnosis; accessible sites including skin, conjunctiva, liver and peripheral lymph nodes give the best yield.

The major differential diagnoses include malignancy (lymphoma), autoimmune lymphoproliferative syndrome, and other granulomatous disorders such as cat-scratch disease, tuberculosis and immunodeficiency.

Treatment of sarcoidosis depends upon the organ involved and the degree of involvement. Isolated lymphadenopathy or mild asymptomatic pulmonary involvement does not require specific systemic treatment. However, most cases require corticosteroid treatment, usually with a steroid sparing agent such as methotrexate or azathioprine. Occasionally anti-TNF monoclonal antibody treatment may be used, especially with severe uveitis and neurosaroid.

References

1. Mier RJ, Shishov M, Higgins GC, et al. Pediatric-onset mixed connective tissue disease. Rheum Dis Clin N Am. 2005;31:483–96.
2. Tsai YY, Yang YH, Yu HH, et al. Fifteen-year experience of pediatric-onset mixed connective tissue disease. Clin Rheumatol. 2010;29:53–8.
3. Michels H. Course of mixed connective tissue disease in children. Ann Med. 1997;29:359–64.
4. Cimaz R, Casadei A, Rose C, et al. Primary Sjögren's syndrome in the paediatric age: a multicentre survey. Eur J Pediatr. 2003;162:661–5.
5. Shiboski SC, Shiboski CH, Criswell L, et al. American College of Rheumatology classification criteria for Sjögren's syndrome: a data-driven, expert consensus approach in the Sjögren's International Collaborative Clinical Alliance cohort. Arthritis Care Res (Hoboken). 2012;63:475–87.
6. Liberman SM. Childhood Sjogren syndrome: insights from adults and animal modes. Curr Opin Rheumatol. 2013;25:651–7.
7. Barukkova J, Sediva A, Vencovsky J, et al. Primary Sjögren's syndrome in children and adolescents: proposal for diagnostic criteria. Clin Exp Rheumatol. 1999;17:381–6.
8. Baszis K, Toib D, Cooper M, et al. Recurrent parotitis as a presentation of primary pediatric Sjögren syndrome. Pediatrics. 2012;129:e179–82.
9. Matsui Y, Takenouchi T, Narabayashi A, et al. Childhood Sjögren syndrome presenting as acute brainstem encephalitis. Brain Dev. 2016;38:158–62.
10. Kamisawa T, Zen Y, Pillai S, Stone JH. IgG4-related disease. Lancet. 2015;385:1460–71.
11. Valeyre D, Prasse A, Nunes H, Uzunhan Y, Brillet PY, Müller-Quernheim J. Sarcoidosis. Lancet. 2014;383:1155–67.

Chapter 8
Vasculitis

8.1   Introduction

Vasculitis is an inflammatory and often destructive process of the blood vessel wall. The vasculitides are difficult to diagnose as presenting symptoms can be nonspecific and multiple organs are involved [1]. Primary vasculitis denotes inflammation of the blood vessels not associated with other inflammatory disease processes. Most vasculitidies are rare in childhood with the exception of Kawasaki disease (KD) and IgA vasculitis (Henoch-Schönlein purpura (HSP)) [2]. Many childhood multisystem inflammatory diseases include components of vasculitis and these are designated as secondary vasculitis. These include bacterial and viral infections, autoimmune and autoinflammatory diseases and malignancies. This chapter will concentrate on primary vasculitis. The initial presentation can be fever, other constitutional symptoms, skin rash, musculoskeletal symptoms, unexplained hypertension or an acute medical emergency with multi-organ failure. A classification of childhood vasculitis was developed based on international consensus, because, childhood onset vasculitis has many unique features compared to adult forms (Table 8.1) [3]. This is a modification of the Chapel Hill classification of adult vasculitis [4].

R.M. Laxer et al., *Pediatric Rheumatology in Clinical Practice*,   141
DOI 10.1007/978-3-319-13099-6_8,
© Springer-Verlag London 2016

TABLE 8.1 Classification of childhood vasculitis [3]

Predominantly large vessel vasculitis

   Takayasu arteritis

Predominantly medium-sized vessel vasculitis

   Childhood polyarteritis nodosa (PAN)

   Cutaneous polyarteritis

   Deficiency of adenosine deaminase 2 (DADA2)

   Kawasaki disease

Predominantly small vessel vasculitis

   Granulomatous

      Granulomatosis with polyangiitis (Wegener)

      Eosinophilic granulomatosis with polyangiitis (Churg-Strauss syndrome)

   Nongranulomatous

      Microscopic polyangiitis

      IgA vasculitis (Henoch-Schönlein purpura)

      Isolated cutaneous leukocytoclastic vasculitis

      Hypocomplementic urticarial vasculitis

Other vasculitides

   Behçet disease

   Vasculitis secondary to infection (including Hepatitis B-associated PAN), malignancies and drugs, including hypersensitivity vasculitis

   Vasculitis associated with connective tissue diseases

   Isolated vasculitis of the central nervous system

   Cogan syndrome

   Unclassified

With permission from BMJ Publishing Group Ltd

8.2 IgA Vasculitis (Henoch-Schönlein Purpura)

8.2.1 Definition

This is a small vessel leukocytoclastic vasculitis, associated with immunoglobulin A deposition in the small vessels of skin and kidneys (Table 8.2) [5].

8.2.2 Epidemiology

This is the most common vasculitis in children, with an incidence between 10 and 20 per 100,000 children [2]. It is more common in boys (1.2:1) with a peak age between 4 and 7 years. Most cases occur in the autumn and winter.

8.2.3 Etiology

Approximately 50 % of cases are preceded by an upper respiratory infection. Many organisms have been implicated, with approximately 33 % of cases following a streptococcal

TABLE 8.2 Classification criteria for IgA vasculitis (Henoch-Schönlein purpura) [5]

Palpable purpura (mandatory criterion) plus 1 of the following criteria:
Abdominal pain
Skin biopsy showing leukocytoclastic vasculitis with predominant IgA deposition or renal biopsy with mesangial proliferative glomerulonephritis
Arthritis or arthralgia
Renal involvement (hematuria and/or proteinuria)

infection [1]. Familial Mediterranean fever (FMF) and complement deficiencies are also associated with this vasculitis.

8.2.4   Clinical Manifestation

Most children present with palpable purpura, predominately in the lower limbs (Fig. 8.1), but it can also involve the upper limbs and face. Occasionally, the rash is edematous (especially in younger patients) and can have superficial ulcerations. Common additional symptoms include arthralgia and arthritis (40–80 %), and colicky abdominal pain (50–75 %),

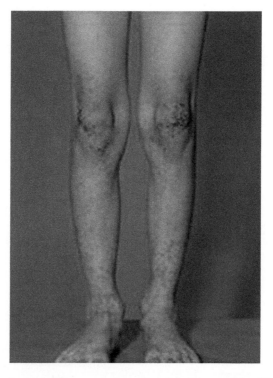

FIGURE 8.1 Palpable purpuric rash of IgA vasculitis (Henoch-Schönlein purpura)

which can be severe. Patients may present with a bloody diarrhea. Ileo-ileal intussusception occurs in <2 %. Renal involvement almost always occurs within 3 months of onset and is seen in nearly half the patients. It usually presents with microscopic hematuria and mild proteinuria but some patients develop nephrotic syndrome, a decrease in renal function and hypertension (sometimes isolated). Other symptoms include orchitis (7–27 % of males) and rarely encephalopathy, pulmonary and cardiac involvements.

8.2.5   Laboratory Findings

The acute phase reactants are normal or only moderately increased. Platelet counts are normal or elevated. About half will have raised serum IgA. Renal involvement is detectable as microscopic hematuria and proteinuria. Occult blood may be found in the stool. ANA and ANCA are negative (or false positive for the latter).

8.2.6   Diagnosis

Palpable purpura, in a dependent fashion, colicky abdominal pain and hematuria/proteinuria establish the diagnosis (Table 8.2). A skin biopsy, if obtained, will show leukocytoclastic vasculitis with immunoflorescence showing a predominant IgA deposition. Renal biopsy is recommended if there is persistent significant proteinuria or a decrease in renal function. Typical findings show deposition of IgA in the mesangium and in severe cases crescentic proliferation. Abdominal ultrasound is warranted if intussusception is suspected.

8.2.7   Treatment and Prognosis

NSAIDs are usually sufficient for symptomatic treatment of joint pain but should be avoided if nephritis is present and other analgesics should be used. Corticosteroids are helpful for severe abdominal pain, edema (orchitis), necrotic skin rashes and arthritis. Whether corticosteroids alter the development and outcome of renal disease is controversial, with most recent studies showing no benefit [6–8]. Corticosteroids are often started intravenously due to abdominal edema. Once given, they should be weaned slowly over 3–4 weeks due to the possibility of a rebound effect if weaned rapidly. In the event of severe nephritis combined corticosteroid and immunosuppressive medication is indicated, although there are no evidence based protocols for the optimal regimen. The disease is mostly self-limiting, lasting up to 12 weeks. Recurrences may occur in up to 25 % of patients. One to 3 % of children develop end stage renal disease, compared to 10–20 % in adults. Mortality is exceedingly rare (0.12–0.7 %) during the acute phase of disease.

8.3   Leukocytoclastic/Hypersensitivity Vasculitis

8.3.1   Definition

This group is defined by the histological picture of leukocyte infiltration of the walls of small blood vessels. It is confined to the skin.

8.3.2   Epidemiology

Unknown, usually affecting older children than those with IgA vasculitis.

8.3.3   Etiology

The causes are diverse, and there may be hypersensitivity reactions, for example, to infections or drugs, most commonly penicillins or cefaclor. It can also be idiopathic.

8.3.4   Clinical Manifestations

In the event of hypersensitivity, symptoms occur 7–14 days after the exposure. Leukocytoclastic vasculitis usually presents with a palpable purpuric skin rash (like IgA vasculitis) with occasional fever, polyarthralgia or even frank arthritis. The rash may be purpuric, urticarial, bullae, livedo, or ecchymotic, and is usually distributed symmetrically, predominantly over the lower legs, but is more likely than IgA vasculitis to involve the trunk.

8.3.5   Laboratory Findings

Mildly increased acute phase reactants are frequently seen. There is occasional eosinophilia and hematuria. Rarely there are decreased levels of serum complement.

8.3.6   Diagnosis

Skin biopsy is the gold standard for diagnosis, as the histological appearance is typical showing leukocytoclastic vasculitis. Venules and capillaries are the most commonly affected blood vessels.

8.3.7   Treatment and Prognosis

Treatment is symptomatic. Removal of the inciting factor, if identified, is crucial. NSAIDs, antihistamines or a short course of corticosteroids usually leads to complete recovery. In recurrent cases various treatments have been used anecdotally, including monthly IV immunoglobulin (IVIG) infusions and colchicine. If the attacks are mild, no treatment is preferred, since the prognosis is excellent.

8.4   Kawasaki Disease (KD)

8.4.1   Definition

This is a multisystem vasculitis first described by Tomisaku Kawasaki in 1967, mainly affecting children under 5 years of age with high fevers, typical skin and mucous membrane involvement and peeling of skin from extremities. The vessels involved are mostly medium sized arteries and, characteristically, produce coronary artery aneurysms. Table 8.3 shows the diagnostic criteria for KD [3].

8.4.2   Epidemiology

KD occurs most frequently in Japanese and Koreans between 1 and 3 years old. Current estimates report an incidence of >250 per 100,000 in Japanese children under 5 years of age and 5–20 per 100,000 among U.S. Caucasians [2, 9]. Among Japanese, there are ~2 % familial occurrence in siblings. It is

TABLE 8.3 Diagnostic criteria for Kawasaki disease [3] (With permission from BMJ Publishing Group Ltd)

Fever persisting for at least 5 days plus 4[a] of the following criteria:
Changes in peripheral extremities or perineal area
Polymorphous exanthema
Bilateral conjunctival injection
Changes of lips and oral cavity: injection of oral and pharyngeal mucosa
Cervical lymphadenopathy

[a]In the presence of coronary artery involvement detected on echocardiography and fever, fewer than 4 of the remaining 5 criteria are sufficient

about 1.5 times more common in boys. Most cases occur in the winter and early spring [10].

8.4.3 Etiology

Often there is a history of a preceding infection, with diverse organisms implicated. The fact that KD occurs as seasonal epidemics supports an infectious trigger with a prolonged reactive inflammatory response. The pathogenesis of conventional antigen vs. superantigen activation of T lymphocytes is highly debated. There are several polymorphisms in immune regulatory genes found mainly among Japanese associated with an increased risk of KD. More recently it was suggested that the innate immune system may play an important role in pathogenesis.

8.4.4 Clinical Manifestations

Patients present with high remitting fevers for over 1 week (when untreated), inflammation of the mucous membranes leading to non-exudative conjunctival injection (with limbic sparing), red tongue, and lip fissuring (Fig. 8.2). Also included in the diagnostic criteria are swelling and redness of the hands and feet, a nonspecific polymorphic skin rash and cervical lymphadenopathy (usually unilateral, the least common occurring of the diagnostic criteria). The child is highly irritable. Joint pains are common. Features suggesting an upper respiratory tract infection, as well as diarrhea, vomiting, ileus, jaundice, hydrops of the gallbladder, pancreatitis, dysuria, pneumonitis, uveitis, convulsions and meningitis can be seen. Cardiac involvement includes myocarditis, pericarditis, tamponade and myocardial infarction. Infrequently, signs of macrophage activation syndrome (see Chap. 3) may be present at disease onset. Perianal peeling can be seen. Periungual skin desquamation and nail changes (Beau lines) are seen after the acute phase. Arthritis may also occur after the acute phase.

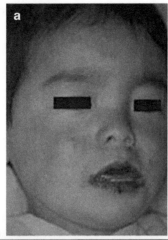

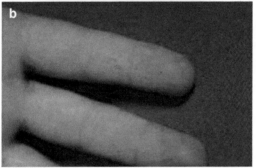

Figure 8.2 (**a**) Kawasaki disease (KD) showing facial rash and mucocutaneous erythema and fissuring. (**b**) Skin desquamation of fingertips in KD

8.4.5   Laboratory Findings

There is a significant elevation in the acute phase reactants. Marked thrombocytosis often occurs as the fever resolves. Sterile pyuria is common but the urine leukocyte esterase test is negative since the pyuria is due to monocytes. Antinuclear antibodies are negative and serum complement is usually normal or elevated. Echocardiography shows coronary artery dilations (Z-score) and aneurysms (Fig. 8.3) in over a quarter of untreated cases 3 to 6 weeks after onset although myocarditis and pericarditis may be seen much earlier.

8.4.6 Diagnosis

Early diagnosis and treatment is essential, because of the risk of coronary artery aneurysms. Differential diagnoses include infections, drug reactions, and other rheumatologic diseases, such as systemic JIA, reactive arthritis, and other vasculitidies. An echocardiogram and ECG are essential if KD is suspected. Incomplete or atypical KD has been described by clinicians if five criteria are not met, and should be suspected particularly in children younger than 1 and older than 6 years of age. All infants under 6 months of age with unexplained fever lasting >1 week need to undergo an echocardiograph, even with no accompanying symptoms [10].

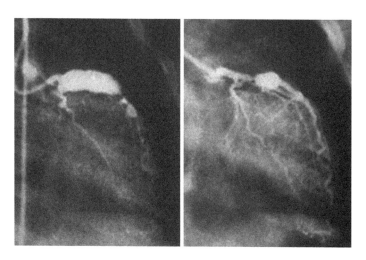

FIGURE 8.3 Coronary artery aneurysms in KD on angiography

8.4.7   Treatment

Children with suspected KD should be admitted to hospital. Once the diagnosis has been made, IVIG (2 g/kg) should be given over 12 h, with aspirin (varying doses are recommended; the American Heart Association recommends 80–100 mg/kg/day). Once afebrile, low dose aspirin is continued (5 mg/kg/day) for 2 months if the echocardiogram is normal. In about 10–15 % symptoms fail to respond, or return 24–36 h after the first dose of IVIG. Approximately two thirds of patients will respond to retreatment [10]. Corticosteroids may be added at this stage, especially in patients with coronary abnormalities, even if minor. Corticosteroid administration of IV methylprednisolone (1 mg/kg twice daily, with some giving an initial pulse of 30 mg/kg), followed by oral prednisolone should be continued until clinical signs of disease activity abate and then weaned (usually over 2 weeks). Anti-TNF agents are used in resistant cases, although the effect on coronary outcomes is still unclear [11]. Aspirin, other anti-platelet agents and anticoagulation in large/giant aneurysms, should be continued in patients with residual coronary artery abnormalities.

8.4.8   Outcome

The disease is usually monocyclic, although recurrence has been reported in ~3 % of Japanese patients. The majority of patients with KD, without coronary aneurysms, recover fully. The acute mortality rate with IVIG treatment is <1 %. Children with coronary artery involvement have an increased risk of coronary heart disease in adult life and will need long-term cardiac care [10].

8.5   Polyarteritis Nodosa (PAN)

8.5.1   Definition

Polyarteritis nodosa is a systemic vasculitis characterized and defined by a typical histological appearance of necrotizing inflammatory changes in medium and/or smaller sized arteries. Table 8.4 shows the pediatric classification criteria for PAN [5].

8.5.2   Epidemiology

Polyarteritis nodosa is a rare vasculitis in childhood, with a mean age of onset of around 9 years. The incidence appears equal in both sexes [12].

TABLE 8.4 Classification criteria for childhood polyarteritis nodosa (PAN) [5]

The presence of (a mandatory criterion):
Biopsy showing small and midsize artery necrotizing vasculitis or angiographic abnormalities[a] (aneurysms, stenosis or occlusions)
And the presence of at least one of the following criteria:
Skin involvement (livedo reticularis, tender subcutaneous nodules, other vasculitic lesions)
Myalgia or muscle tenderness
Systemic hypertension, relative to childhood normative data
Mononeuropathy or polyneuropathy
Abnormal urinalysis and/or impaired renal function

[a]Should include formal angiography if MRA or CT angiography is negative

8.5.3   Etiology

Childhood onset PAN can be a single acute episode following an infectious trigger, or a relapsing disease that has no obvious infectious or other external triggers. It has been associated with streptococcal infection [13]. Unlike adults, there are only rare cases associated with hepatitis B infection even prior to widespread hepatitis B vaccination. An autosomal recessive PAN like vasculopathy caused by from mutations in the *CECR1* gene encoding adenosine deaminase 2 (DADA2) was discovered, mainly in patients from Georgian Jewish origin [14]. PAN is also associated with familial Mediterranean fever (FMF), usually with a milder course than idiopathic disease [15].

8.5.4   Clinical Manifestations

PAN presents with constitutional features (95 %) of fever, lethargy and weight loss, skin rash (50–60 %), including painful palpable purpura and nodules, livedo reticularis (Fig. 8.4), ecchymosis, ulcers and gangrene. Arthralgia/myalgia (50–60 %), especially calf pain, abdominal pain (67 %), testicular

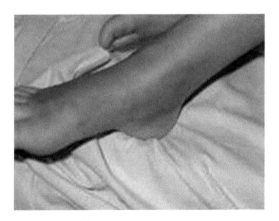

FIGURE 8.4 Livedo rash of polyarteritis nodosa (PAN)

pain and headaches are common. There is often evidence of renovascular involvement (up to 80 %), e.g., hypertension, neurological involvement (40 %), especially mononeuritis multiplex, cardiovascular involvement (45 %) and, rarely cough/hemoptysis. There may be coronary artery involvement. In the DADA2 variant, strokes, including hemorrhagic, are common. Perirenal hematoma is characteristic of FMF-associated PAN.

8.5.5   Laboratory Findings

Patients have raised acute phase reactants and anemia of chronic disease. Autoantibodies, such as ANCA, are usually absent. Other abnormal tests will depend on the affected organ system.

Skin and other organ biopsies (e.g. muscle, sural nerve) show fibrinoid necrotizing vasculitis, mainly in medium or small muscular arteries, often segmental (Fig. 8.5).

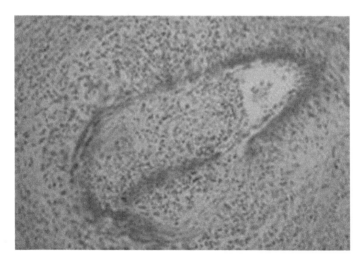

FIGURE 8.5 Histology of necrotizing vasculitis of medium sized artery in PAN

Arteriographic demonstration of aneurysms of medium-sized arteries in a beading pattern, especially at bifurcation points in the celiac, superior and inferior mesenteric and renal arteries, is the radiologic diagnostic gold standard (Fig. 8.6). MRA or CT angiography is often not sufficiently sensitive for the size of the vessels involved.

8.5.6   Diagnosis

Any child with fever of unknown origin, irritability, myalgia, weight loss and unexplained multiple system involvement should have a vasculitis workup. This consists of exclusion of infectious causes of fever and other types of multisystem inflammatory diseases. Diagnosis is supported by the demonstration of acute phase reactants along with abnormal tests for specific organ function and, ultimately, a biopsy, angiogram, or both. In the appropriate ethnicity, or in the event of a stroke, genetic testing for DADA2 mutations should be performed.

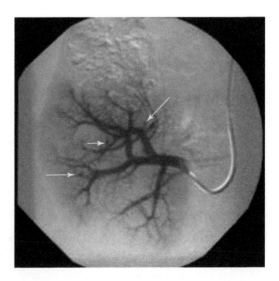

FIGURE 8.6 Aneurysms of the renal arterial axis in PAN (*arrows*)

8.5.7   Treatment

Pharmacological treatment consists of two phases, induction and maintenance. Induction is usually with IV methylprednisolone pulses at 30 mg/kg (maximum 1,000 mg) for 3–5 days followed by oral prednisone (1 mg/kg/day, up to 60 mg/d). Cyclophosphamide is added for significant gastrointestinal, CNS, renal and cardiac disease and for mononeuritis and is given either orally for 3–6 months at 2 mg/kg/day or IV as fortnightly (15 mg/kg) or monthly pulses of 500–1,000 mg/m^2. A relatively short maintenance therapy primarily using azathioprine (2–2.5 mg/kg/day, up to 150 mg/d) is recommended for between 6 and 12 months. IVIG may be corticosteroid sparing. Plasmapheresis may be useful in hepatitis B related disease. TNF inhibitors are extremely effective in DADA2-related PAN, even in severe cases not responsive to cyclophosphamide. The role of biologics in idiopathic PAN is still not clear.

8.5.8   Outcome

The course of PAN is variable depending on the organs involved. It is usually monocyclic, but can be relapsing in about one third of cases, often with long periods of remission. The outcome, in the largest pediatric retrospective series (N = 110) was much better than reported in adults with only one (1 %) death and two (2 %) with end stage renal disease [12].

8.6   Cutaneous Polyarteritis Nodosa

Cutaneous polyarteritis is characterized by the presence of subcutaneous nodular, painful vasculitic lesions with or without livedo reticularis and no systemic or internal organ involvement, except for myalgia, arthralgia, nonerosive arthritis and occasionally fever. Cutaneous polyarteritis is often associated with serologic or microbiologic evidence of streptococcal infection.

8.6.1   Clinical Features

The rash is raised, red and painful with surrounding tissue edema. It characteristically occurs around the eyes, calves and the instep of the foot (Fig. 8.7). Rashes near the joint often cause periarticular edema and mimic arthritis by causing pain and restriction of motion. The child is usually very irritable.

There have been reports of relapsing cutaneous polyarteritis, evolving into systemic PAN after penicillin prophylaxis was stopped [13].

8.6.2   Laboratory Features

A marked acute phase response is seen. Urinalysis, renal and liver function tests are normal. Autoantibody screen and ANCA

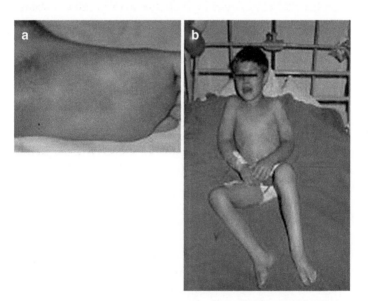

Figure 8.7 (a) Typical palpable, painful rash of cutaneous polyarteritis in the foot instep. (b) A child with cutaneous polyarteritis showing the edematous, raised macular rashes over eyes, arms, and legs

are negative. Patients with poststreptococcal cutaneous PAN have elevated titers of antistreptolysin O and anti-DNase B.

8.6.3   Diagnosis

A deep skin biopsy showing non-granulomatous necrotizing vasculitis of small muscular arteries and the combination of the above clinical and laboratory features confirms diagnosis.

8.6.4   Treatment

Corticosteroids abort the inflammatory changes within 1–2 weeks. The steroid dose can then be tapered over the next few (up to 6) months. Relapses usually occur if this reduction is too fast. Prophylactic penicillin should be given in cases where there is demonstrable recent streptococcal infection, similar to rheumatic fever protocols.

8.6.5   Outcome

The course of cutaneous polyarteritis is usually benign. Most patients recover after a course of corticosteroid therapy. A relapsing course suggests evolution to systemic PAN [13].

8.7   Granulomatosis with Polyangiitis (Wegener): GPA

8.7.1   Definition

This is a necrotizing granulomatous vasculitis, mainly affecting small and medium size blood vessels of the upper and lower respiratory tracts and kidneys. Table 8.5 shows the pediatric classification criteria for GPA [5].

TABLE 8.5 Classification criteria for granulomatosis with polyangiitis (Wegener) [5]

The presence of 3 of the following 6 criteria:

Renal involvement – abnormal urinalysis/biopsy[a]

Granulomatous inflammation/vasculitis on biopsy

Nasal-sinus inflammation

Laryngeal, subglottic, tracheal, or endobronchial stenosis

Abnormal chest radiograph or CT

Proteinase 3- antineutrophil cytoplasmic antibody (ANCA) or C-ANCA staining

[a]If kidney biopsy is performed, it characteristically shows necrotizing pauci-immune glomerulonephritis, often crescentic

8.7.2   Epidemiology

GPA is rare in children (1–2 per 1,000,000 per year), mainly affecting older children [16]. Four of the largest series have described 130 children with GPA [17]. In children, unlike adults, females are affected more frequently [16].

8.7.3   Etiology

Although the etiology is unknown, it is clear that antineutrophil cytoplasmic antibodies (ANCA) play a pathogenic role in the disease.

8.7.4   Clinical Manifestations

Patients often present with fever, malaise and weight loss (90–95 %). Other common nonspecific features include arthralgia/arthritis (55–65 %) and nodular, purpuric (occasionally ulcerative) skin rashes (25–50 %). More specifically, 80–90 % (20 % as presenting symptom) have upper respiratory involvement. This may include chronic rhinorrhea, epistaxis, nasal crusting and ulcerations, sinusitis and otitis media, the latter two unresponsive to antibiotics. Collapse of the nasal bridge is a common sign of damage (Fig. 8.8). Subglottic stenosis manifest by stridor, hoarseness and respiratory distress is seen more frequently (up to 40 %) and has more clinical significance in children than adults (Fig. 8.9). Lower respiratory symptoms (80–90 %) include cough, dyspnea and hemoptysis. Hematuria and proteinuria, with or without hypertension, indicates renal involvement (80–90 %). Some patients develop rapidly progressive glomerulonephritis with deteriorating renal function. Eye manifestations (35–55 %) include pseudotumor, proptosis of the orbit, scleritis and uveitis. Hearing can be impaired. Peripheral neuropathy may develop in up to 25 % of children. Pulmonary embolism and other vascular thromboses occur in about 10 % of patients with GPA.

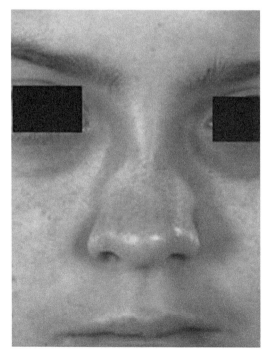

FIGURE 8.8 Typical saddle shaped nose of granulomatosis with polyangiitis (Wegener)

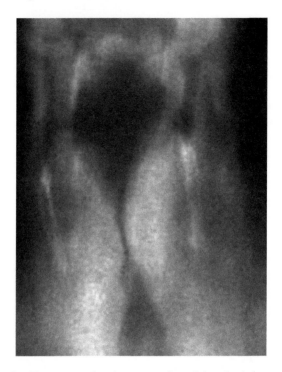

FIGURE 8.9 Tomogram showing narrowing of the glottis by granulomatous tissue

8.7.5   Laboratory Findings

There is evidence of an acute phase response. In addition, ANCA is usually present in the serum (>90 %), primarily with a cytoplasmic pattern (c-ANCA), mainly directed against serine proteinase 3 (PR3). There is debate whether ANCA titers need to be monitored to determine treatment efficacy or predict the development of a relapse. Absence of ANCA is usually evidence against a flare but not vice versa.

Urinalysis, chest radiographs and high resolution CT (the latter more sensitive) and sinus CT demonstrates systemic involvement. Chest imaging shows pneumonitis, shadowing indicating alveolar infiltration and nodules, often cavitary

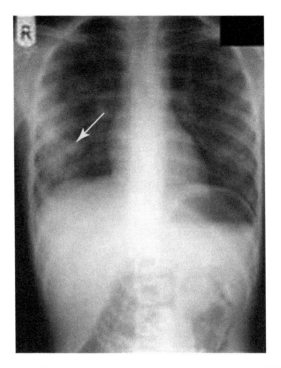

FIGURE 8.10 Chest x-ray showing nodule (*arrow*) in a child with granulomatosis with polyangiitis (Wegener)

(Fig. 8.10). Laryngoscopy or tomography/CT can demonstrate subglottic stenosis (Fig. 8.9). Monitoring pulmonary function with DLCO (increased with pulmonary hemorrhage) can be useful. Typically, the histology of the lung lesions shows a necrotizing vasculitis with granulomata. Nasal and sinus biopsy usually show only non-specific inflammation. Kidney biopsy demonstrates pauci-immune glomerulonephritis with crescentic proliferation.

8.7.6 Diagnosis

The triad of upper and lower respiratory tract and kidney involvement with c-ANCA (anti-PR3) antibodies is diagnostic.

In classic cases with positive antibodies tissue biopsy is not necessary for diagnosis. Upper airway involvement distinguishes GPA from microscopic polyangiitis. The latter is nongranulomatous and usually has positive p-ANCA (anti-myeloperoxidase) antibodies. Limited GPA can exist without lower respiratory and renal lesions. Other causes of pulmonary-renal syndrome, such as SLE and anti-basement membrane antibody (Goodpasture) disease should be excluded.

8.7.7   Treatment

Induction treatment of moderate to severe disease includes use of prednisone (1 mg/kg/day, often with IV methylprednisolone pulses initially) and cyclophosphamide (various protocols, see Sect. 8.5.7) or rituximab, the latter especially in females of child bearing capacity. Milder disease can be treated with methotrexate or azathioprine in addition to prednisone. Plasmapheresis may be beneficial in patients with rapidly progressive renal dysfunction or pulmonary hemorrhage or those with features of microangiopathy with clots. Maintenance therapy following remission induction (usually after 3 months of cyclophosphamide therapy) includes use of azathioprine (preferred), mycophenolate or methotrexate, usually for up to 2 years. There is debate regarding the length of corticosteroid therapy; there is some evidence that very long-term therapy, even at low doses, may prevent disease flares. It is possible that the use of rituximab reduces the need for maintenance therapy. Rituximab is preferred to cyclophosphamide for treatment of disease flares. There is no clear evidence that using trimethoprim/sulfamethoxazole is effective, although often used to prevent *Pneumocystis jirovecii* infection and likely indicated if recurrent upper airway infection is a problem. Subglottic stenosis is treated primary by local/topical therapy with corticosteroid and mitomycin injections and dilatations.

8.7.8   Outcome

In approximately 50 % the disease may relapse thus requiring regular follow-up by a rheumatologist, otolaryngologist, pulmonologist and nephrologist. The 5-year mortality rate is less than 5 %.

8.8   Microscopic Polyangiitis

This is a necrotizing pauci-immune vasculitis affecting small vessels and often associated with a high titer of perinuclear ANCA (p-ANCA), due to antibodies to myeloperoxidase (MPO). Necrotizing glomerulonephritis is very common, as is pulmonary capillaritis without granulomatous lesions of the respiratory tract. Contrary to GPA, the upper respiratory tract is spared.

8.8.1   Clinical Features

The presenting pulmonary symptoms are often acute, with pneumonitis, hemoptysis, fever and malaise. Rapidly progressive renal failure with features of nephritic and nephrotic syndrome may occur, as well as cutaneous features of palpable purpuric lesions.

8.8.2   Laboratory Features

See GPA. The pattern of antibodies is usually a p-ANCA pattern, with specificity to MPO.

8.8.3   Diagnosis

See GPA. A renal biopsy is often necessary to differentiate between causes of lung-renal syndromes.

8.8.4   Treatment

Similar to GPA.

8.8.5   Outcome

Similar to GPA, although disease flares are less frequent.

8.9   Eosinophilic Granulomatosis with Polyangiitis (Churg-Strauss Syndrome)

This is an eosinophilic-rich and granulomatous necrotizing pauci-immune vasculitis affecting small to medium size vessels. It is very rare in childhood and the cause is unknown [18].

8.9.1   Clinical Features

Children usually present with years of treatment resistant asthma, allergic rhinitis and nasal polyposis with eosinophilia. Later patients can develop pneumonia, hemoptysis, fever and malaise. Mononeuritis multiplex is common (55–70 %) and papular rashes are apparent in 50–67 %. Cardiac involvement is more common (25–45 %) than in other ANCA-related vasculitidies. On the other hand renal involvement is less common (about 20 %). Musculoskeletal symptoms are common.

8.9.2   Laboratory Features

Eosinophilia is almost university seen with counts as high as 30,000/mm^3. ANCA, most commonly p-ANCA with MPO specificity, is seen in a minority of children.

8.9.3   Diagnosis

Chest imaging usually shows transient pulmonary/alveolar infiltrates with a fluffy and patchy character. Cardiac (MRI) and sinus imaging may be helpful. Pulmonary function and nerve conduction tests may be necessary. Skin, lung and nerve biopsies usually confirm the diagnosis with findings of eosinophil infiltrates in vessel walls with fibrinoid necrosis and extravascular necrotizing granulomas.

8.9.4   Treatment

Similar to GPA. Small series have shown the potential efficacy of the anti-IL-5 antibody mepolizumab, anti CD-20 rituximab and anti IgE antibody omalizumab.

8.9.5   Outcome

The outcome has markedly improved with modern therapy with >80 % remission rate and 10 year survival >75 %.

8.10   Takayasu Arteritis

8.10.1   Definition

This is a large vessel granulomatous vasculitis of the aorta, its main branches and pulmonary artery. Post surgical/mortem pathologic specimens most commonly show a mononuclear infiltrate of the vasa vasorum. Table 8.6 shows the pediatric classification for Takayasu arteritis (TA) [5].

8.10.2   Epidemiology

TA is seen most frequently in females (in children >70 %) and in patients of Far East origin. However it can be seen in

TABLE 8.6 Classification criteria for Takayasu arteritis [5]

Angiographic abnormalities of the aorta or its main branches and pulmonary artery (mandatory criterion) plus 1 of the following criteria:
Absent peripheral pulses or claudication
Blood pressure discrepancy in any limb
Bruits
Hypertension
Elevated acute phase reactants

all ethnicities. The onset in children is usually during adolescence [19, 20].

8.10.3   Etiology

The cause is unknown. However, TA is seen in association with Crohn disease and in the developing countries in association with tuberculosis.

8.10.4   Clinical Features

The classic presentation in children is with constitutional features (~50 %) of fever, fatigue, malaise, weight loss and hypertension (80–90 %). Other common features include headaches (>80 %), dizziness, syncope, back and abdominal pain and angina. Limb claudication is less common in children. Myocardial infarction and stroke may occur. Although pulmonary artery involvement is common, pulmonary symptoms are rare. Some children present late in the course with hypertension alone and no history of a preceding unexplained inflammatory illness. Physical findings include diminished peripheral pulses, bruits over large arteries and blood pressure asymmetry between limbs. Late complications of hypertension include retinal changes and cardiomyopathy.

8.10.5   Laboratory Features

Acute phase reactant elevation is almost universal in the initial phases and often helpful in following the disease course. However, there are many cases of disease progression despite normal acute phase reactants. There are no specific autoantibodies detected.

8.10.6   Diagnosis and Imaging

Early suspicion of TA is difficult due to the non-specific symptoms in most patients. However, the triad of systemic symptoms, hypertension and acute phase reactant elevation is classic. When suspected, large vessel imaging of the aorta and its main branches by formal angiography, MRI/MRA or CT angiography is diagnostic (Fig. 8.11). These may demonstrate vessel wall thickening/edema, stenoses, occlusions and aneurysms (the latter is more common in the Far East). Periodic imaging is crucial in following the disease progression. The role of fluorodeoxyglucose PET scans in demonstrating active inflammation in vessel walls is still unclear. Other diseases that can involve large and medium sized vessels such as fibromuscular dysplasia and disorders of collagen genes must be excluded when there is no history of an associated inflammatory syndrome.

8.10.7   Treatment

Corticosteroids are the mainstay of therapy but disease relapse is frequent during tapering. Steroid sparing medications, primarily methotrexate, is frequently used. In severe cases cyclophosphamide may be indicated. In frequently relapsing or persistent disease TNF inhibitors (mainly infliximab) or tocilizumab may be beneficial. Aspirin is often recommended and may prevent thrombotic events. Patients may need several medications to control hypertension. Occasionally, vascular repair is needed (percutaneous bal-

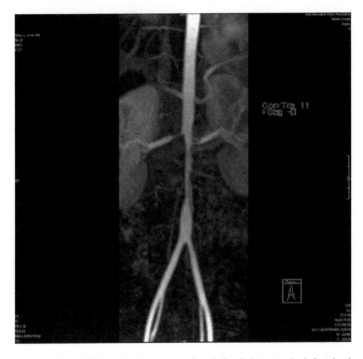

FIGURE 8.11 MRA showing stenosis of the infra-renal abdominal aorta and bilateral proximal renal arteries in a patient with Takayasu arteritis

loon angioplasty or bypass surgery; stents are not recommended in TA), particularly for hypertension, abdominal angina or claudication. Surgical treatment should be deferred to periods of quiescent disease.

8.10.8   Outcome

The disease is monophasic in ~25 % of patient and relapsing in the rest, thus long-term immunosuppressive therapy is needed in the majority of patients. Mortality is rare; however, disease or treatment related morbidity is common.

8.11 Primary Angiitis of the Central Nervous System

8.11.1 Definition

This is a vasculitis confined to the central nervous system (CNS) [21]. In children there are three main subclasses of primary angiitis of the CNS (PACNS).

1. Non-progressive PACNS, usually involving one medium size artery.
2. Progressive angiographic positive PACNS with development of new lesions 3 months after diagnosis. This form involves large to medium sized vessels, is frequently bilateral and involves distal as well as proximal vessels.
3. Angiographic negative PACNS involving small vessels, which is also a progressive disease.

8.11.2 Epidemiology

PACNS is extremely rare in children, the incidence is unknown. In adults, PACNS is more frequent in males. Childhood PACNS is diagnosed at a median of ~10 years of age.

8.11.3 Etiology

The cause is unknown. However, PACNS may be triggered by infections, particularly varicella-zoster.

8.11.4 Clinical Features

Non-progressive and angiographic positive PACNS usually presents with stroke-like symptoms (motor, speech and/or sensory). Angiographic negative small vessel

PACNS presents usually with progressive cognitive and other brain dysfunction, visual deficits, seizures, psychiatric symptoms, headaches and encephalopathy. Children with this subtype may have constitutional symptoms, like fever and malaise.

8.11.5   Laboratory and Imaging Features

Acute phase reactants are usually normal in angiographic positive PACNS but may be elevated in angiographic negative PACNS. In angiographic negative PACNS cerebrospinal fluid usually demonstrates elevated opening pressure and protein levels, and pleocytosis. In both types of PACNS von Willebrand factor related antigen may be elevated. Autoantibodies are usually negative. MRI findings include signs of infarcts as well as high intensity lesions on T2 or FLAIR techniques, enhancing with gadolinium, mainly in the subcortical white and deep grey matter and leptomeninges (Fig. 8.12). Imaging findings in angiographic positive disease shows stenosis, tapering, beading, tortuosity and/or occlusion of large to medium size vessels (Fig. 8.13). Formal angiography may be necessary to demonstrate distal blood vessels, particularly in the posterior circulation. Brain biopsy in children with angiographic negative PACNS demonstrates mostly lymphocytic vasculitis and perivascular infiltrates unlike the granulomatous lesions more common in adults.

8.11.6   Diagnosis

PACNS should be suspected in the differential diagnosis of unexplained neurologic deficits. Inflammatory markers, cerebrospinal fluid analysis, appropriate imaging and a brain biopsy in angiographic negative cases should be part of the work-up.

There is an extensive differential diagnosis of genetic, developmental, infectious, inflammatory, metabolic, prothrombotic and malignant causes that can mimic PACNS.

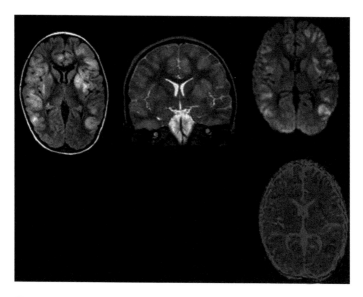

FIGURE 8.12 Brain MRI demonstrating extensive multilobar corti-cal/subcortical and left basal ganglia swelling and signal abnormality with diffusion restriction consistent with small vessel vasculitis. The MRA (not included) was normal (Courtsey of Dr. Helen Branson, The Hospital for Sick Children, Toronto, CA)

8.11.7   Treatment

A multidisciplinary team of neurologists, radiologists and rheumatologists are necessary for managing these patients. Non-progressive PACNS is usually treated with a 3 month course of corticosteroids and anticoagulation. Both types of progressive PACNS are treated with induction therapy of high-dose corticosteroids and cyclophosphamide for 3–6 months, followed by mycophenolate mofetil (preferred) or azathioprine maintenance therapy, usually for up to 2 years.

8.11.8   Outcome

The prognosis has markedly improved with modern therapy, with rare cases of mortality. However morbidity secondary to

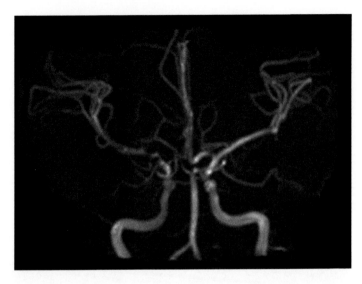

FIGURE 8.13 Brain MRA showing right middle cerebral artery narrowing and irregularity consistent with large vessel vasculitis (Courtsey of Dr. Helen Branson, The Hospital for Sick Children, Toronto, CA)

neurologic deficits prior to treatment can be considerable. Angiographic positive PACNS is mostly monophasic if treated appropriately. Recurrences of angiographic negative disease are reported in ~40 % of patients.

8.12   Behçet Disease (BD)

8.12.1   Definition

A systemic vasculitis, with characteristic oral and genital ulcers, skin lesions, eye, gastrointestinal, nervous system and joint manifestations.

8.12.2   Epidemiology

Behçet disease is more common in ethnic groups from the Far East, along the "Silk-Road" and the Eastern Mediterranean (most commonly Turks). It usually presents in the second and third decade and is rare in children. Both genders are equally affected. Males, however, have a more severe course. A family history may be present in >10 % of pediatric patients [22].

8.12.3   Etiology

HLA B51 has been found to be associated with Turkish and Far East patients with BD, but the etiology remains unclear. Recently, other gene associations have been described, such as in the IL-10 region, IL-12 and 23 receptor regions and STAT and ERAP-1 pathways as well as heterozygous mutations in the *MEFV* (FMF) gene.

8.12.4   Clinical Manifestations

In children recurrent oral ulcerations are almost invariably the first symptom and may precede other manifestations by many years. Oral ulcerations are often multiple, deep and painful. Genital ulcers (~60 %) most commonly occur on the scrotum (males) and the labia (females). Ulcers usually heal over 1–4 weeks. Scarring can occur with deep ulcerations. Skin lesions (55–80 %) can vary from nodular, like erythema nodosum to acneiform, papulopustular or leukocytoclastic vasculitis. The pathergy phenomenon, which is defined as the development of a papular/pustular lesion 24–48 h following a needle prick, is seen mainly among patients of Mediterranean and Far East ancestry (~45 %). Uveitis (30–50 %) is particularly seen in young males and manifests with severe, bilateral, relapsing panuveitis. Retinal vasculitis with edema is frequent.

Thrombosis in both the venous (more common) and arterial systems are common (~33 %). Most frequent are superficial venous thrombosis but deeper veins can be involved as in Budd-Chiari syndrome and sinus vein thrombosis. Pulmonary artery aneurysms and thrombosis are particularly a poor prognostic factor. Japanese patients commonly (rare in Western populations) present with gastrointestinal involvement, predominately ulcers in the ileum and cecum that may perforate. Rectal involvement is rare. Arthralgia and arthritis are common (~50 %). CNS involvement (5–10 %) is a poor prognostic factor.

8.12.5   Laboratory Findings

There are no specific tests other than elevations in acute phase reactants. Imaging may demonstrate some of the vascular complications.

8.12.6   Diagnosis

Classification criteria, proposed by an international study group in 1990, require the presence of recurrent oral ulceration, plus two of the following:

- Recurrent genital ulceration
- Eye lesions (typical panuveitis, or retinal vasculitis)
- Skin lesions (nodular/folliculitis/papulopustular/acneiform/purpura)
- Positive pathergy test (read by physician at 24 h after skin prick)

In addition to the above, the history, examination and appropriate imaging and laboratory tests are important to define the extent of organ involvement and exclude other rheumatic diseases and infections.

8.12.7   Treatment

No controlled studies have been performed in children with BD. Adult studies have shown that colchicine (up to 1.5 mg/day) is effective for mucocutaneous disease with a better response for genital ulcers, erythema nodosum and arthritic manifestations [23]. Topical corticosteroids are useful for mucosal disease and short courses of systemic corticosteroids are occasionally used. Other alternatives include pentoxyfillin, dapsone and thalidomide/lenalidomide for especially resistant mucocutaneous disease. For eye disease azathioprine, cyclosporine and interferon-α-2a may be effective as steroid-sparing medications. More recently anti-TNF antibodies and IL-1 inhibitors have been used. In severe vasculitis organ involvement, pulse IV methylprednisolone and cyclophospha-mide are often employed. Anticoagulation is not effective for treatment of thrombotic events.

8.12.8   Outcome

The disease is characterized by exacerbations and remission and the intensity usually abates over time. However, Behçet disease is a significant cause of mortality, especially due to bleeding pulmonary artery aneurysms [24]. Uveitis can cause blindness, especially in young males.

Other causes of morbidity and mortality are ruptured peripheral aneurysms, severe central nervous system disease, Budd-Chiari syndrome and intestinal ulceration and perfora-tion, which is especially prominent among the Japanese.

References

1. Weiss PF. Pediatric vasculitis. Pediatr Clin North Am. 2012;59:407–23.
2. Gardner-Medwin JM, Dolezalova P, Cummins C, Southwood TR. Incidence of Henoch-Schönlein purpura, Kawasaki disease, and rare vasculitides in children of different ethnic origins. Lancet. 2002;360:1197–202.
3. Ozen S, Ruperto N, Dillon MJ, et al. EULAR/PReS endorsed consensus criteria for the classification of childhood vasculitides. Ann Rheum Dis. 2006;65:936–41.
4. Jennette JC, Falk RJ, Bacon PA, et al. 2012 revised international Chapel Hill consensus conference nomenclature of vasculitides. Arthritis Rheum. 2013;65:1–11.

5. Ozen S, Pistorio A, Iusan SM, et al. EULAR/PRINTO/PRES criteria for Henoch-Schönlein purpura, childhood polyarteritis nodosa, childhood Wegener granulomatosis and childhood Takayasu arteritis: Ankara 2008. Part II: final classification criteria. Ann Rheum Dis. 2010;69:798–806.
6. Chartapisak W, Opastiraku S, Willis NS, et al. Prevention and treatment of renal disease in Henoch-Schönlein purpura: a systematic review. Arch Dis Child. 2009;94:132–7.
7. Zaffanello M, Fanos V. Treatment-based literature of Henoch-Schönlein purpura nephritis in childhood. Pediatr Nephrol. 2009;24:1901–11.
8. Saulsbury FT. Henoch-Schönlein purpura. Curr Opin Rheumatol. 2010;22:598–602.
9. Makino N, Nakamura Y, Yashiro M, et al. Descriptive epidemiology of Kawasaki disease in Japan, 2011–2012: from the results of the 22nd nationwide survey. J Epidemiol. 2015;25:239–45.
10. Newburger JW, Takahashi M, Gerber MA, et al. Diagnosis, treatment, and long-term management of Kawasaki disease: a statement for health professionals from the Committee on Rheumatic Fever, Endocarditis, and Kawasaki Disease, Council on Cardiovascular Disease in the Young American Heart Association. Pediatrics. 2004;114:1708.
11. Sundel RP. Kawasaki disease. Rheum Dis Clin North Am. 2015;41:63–73.
12. Ozen S, Anton J, Arisoy N, et al. Juvenile polyarteritis: results of a multicenter survey of 110 children. J Pediatr. 2004;145:517–22.
13. Díaz-Pérez JL, De Lagrán ZM, Díaz-Ramón JL, Winkelmann RK. Cutaneous polyarteritis nodosa. Semin Cutan Med Surg. 2007;26:77–86.
14. Navon-Elkan P, Pierce SB, Segel R, et al. Mutant adenosine deaminase 2 in a polyarteritis nodosa vasculopathy. N Engl J Med. 2014;370:921–31.
15. Ozen S, Ben-Chetrit E, Bakkaloglu A, et al. Polyarteritis nodosa in patients with familial Mediterranean fever (FMF): a concomitant disease or a feature of FMF? Semin Arthritis Rheum. 2001;30:281–7.
16. Cabral DA, Uribe AG, Benseler S, ARChiVe (A Registry for Childhood Vasculitis: e-entry) Investigators Network, et al. Classification, presentation, and initial treatment of Wegener's granulomatosis in childhood. Arthritis Rheum. 2009;60:3413–24.
17. Twilt M, Benseler S. Childhood antineutrophil cytoplasmic antibodies associated vasculitides. Curr Opin Rheumatol. 2014;26:50–5.

18. Gendelman S, Zeft A, Spalding SJ. Childhood-onset eosinophilic granulomatosis with polyangiitis (formerly Churg-Strauss syndrome): a contemporary single-center cohort. J Rheumatol. 2013;40:929–35.
19. Brunner J, Feldman BM, Tyrrell PN, et al. Takayasu arteritis in children and adolescents. Rheumatology (Oxford). 2010;49: 1806–14.
20. Szugye HS, Zeft AS, Spalding SJ. Takayasu arteritis in the pediatric population: a contemporary United States-based single center cohort. Pediatr Rheumatol Online J. 2014;12:21.
21. Twilt M, Benseler SM. The spectrum of CNS vasculitis in children and adults. Nat Rev Rheumatol. 2011;8:97–107.
22. Koné-Paut I, Darce-Bello M, Shahram F, et al. Paediatric Behçet's disease: an international cohort study of 110 patients. One-year follow-up data. Rheumatology (Oxford). 2011;50: 184–8.
23. Hatemi G, Silman A, et al. EULAR recommendations for the management of Behçet disease. Ann Rheum Dis. 2008;67: 1656–62.
24. Yazici H, Basaran G, Hamuryudan V, et al. The ten-year mortality in Behcet's syndrome. Br J Rheumatol. 1996;35:139–41.

Chapter 9
Lyme Arthritis

9.1 Introduction

Steere et al. discovered Lyme disease in the 1970s while investigating an outbreak of childhood arthritis in Old Lyme, Connecticut [1]. It was subsequently found to be due to a tick borne spirochete, *Borrelia burgdorferi*.

9.2 Definition

Lyme disease is characterised by a flu-like illness followed by cutaneous disease (erythema migrans), and then, in some, neurologic (Bell palsy, meningitis, radiculoneuropathy, and encephalopathy), cardiac (heart block and congestive heart failure) or arthritis; all due to B. burgdorferi [2].

9.3 Epidemiology

Lyme arthritis is limited to the Northern Hemisphere in temperate regions where the vector is found, generally in central Europe (although it is described throughout the entire European continent) and in North America, especially in the northeastern United States and northern Midwest. It is rare in Asia. It occurs equally in boys and girls and has been

R.M. Laxer et al., *Pediatric Rheumatology in Clinical Practice*,   181
DOI 10.1007/978-3-319-13099-6_9,
© Springer-Verlag London 2016

reported in children of all ages, especially in those exposed to ticks (children who play in the woods and young adults who hike or camp).

9.4   Etiology

Lyme disease results from an infection with the spirochete B. burgdorferi in North America and in Europe B. garinii and afzelii that is transmitted by an Ixodes tick. This is a very small tick (about the size of head of pin), not the wood tick more frequently found on pets. The primary reservoir for the organism is white-footed mice, voles, and deer; humans are incidental hosts.

9.5   Clinical Manifestations

The tick prefers to feed in warm moist areas so the bite usually occurs in the groin, axilla, breast, and neck. It is at this site, 1–2 weeks later, that the initial rash will develop. It is a painless enlarging annular lesion that clears centrally as it enlarges peripherally giving it a ring-like appearance, known as erythema migrans (Fig. 9.1). Flu-like symptoms may accompany the rash. The next most common manifestation is arthritis that will follow the rash by weeks to months and is typically a monarthritis of the knee with massive swelling, frequently without pain (Fig. 9.2). The arthritis lasts a few days or weeks and completely resolves, but may recur weeks to months later. About two-thirds of the patients with arthritis have an oligoarthritis pattern of joint involvement (overwhelmingly a single knee) and only rarely is it polyarticular. Other, less common features are Bell palsy, encephalitis, uveitis, carditis, and heart block. Neurological involvement can occur, but not in the absence of prior characteristic Lyme disease manifestations [3].

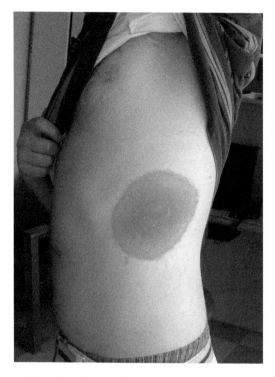

FIGURE 9.1 Typical erythema migrans showing the expanding target lesion

9.6 Laboratory Features

The IgM antibody response to the Lyme spirochete peaks 2–6 weeks after infection and disappears within another month. The IgM peak is followed by prolonged IgG antibody production. Initially, screening for both IgM and IgG done by enzyme immunosorbent assay (EIA) or immunofluorescence assay (IFA) for these antibodies should be obtained. However, these are fraught with false positives so all positive or equivocal tests should be confirmed with Western Blot

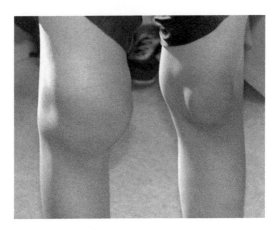

FIGURE 9.2 Massive painless effusion in a child with Lyme arthritis

testing for specific antibody production against different spirochetal outer surface proteins (Osp). IgM antibodies against two of three Osp are confirmatory of recent infection; most of these children will also have positive IgG antibodies to five of ten Osp bands. Virtually all patients have an antibody response to the spirochete [2]. The ANA and RF tests are negative.

Synovial fluid is inflammatory with an average of 25,000 white blood cells per cm [3, 4]. PCR of the synovial fluid may help in isolated patients in whom the diagnosis is not readily apparent, although it generally is not needed.

9.7   Establishing the Diagnosis

The diagnosis of Lyme arthritis is generally straightforward, even if there is no history of tick bite and rash but reasonable temporal and geographic exposure to the tick. The joint is massively swollen with little pain. The synovial fluid is inflammatory. Testing for both IgG and IgM antibodies reveal a positive screen by EIA or IFA and is confirmed by

Western blot testing with at least 2–3 IgM positive bands and 5–10 IgG positive bands [2–4].

9.8   Treatment

Lyme arthritis is usually successfully treated with doxycycline 100 mg orally twice daily for 2–4 weeks, or amoxicillin 500 mg or 17 mg/kg three times daily for 3–4 weeks in children less than 9 years of age or in pregnant women since doxycycline will stain enamel in the forming tooth [5]. Cefuroxime axetil is a better alternative for the penicillin allergic, since macrolides (including erythromycin and azithromycin) are clinically less effective. Occasionally, intravenous ceftriaxone may be necessary if the initial treatment fails. Jarisch–Herxheimer-like reactions may occur after starting therapy, mostly manifest by fever and arthralgias. See Table 9.1 for treatment alternatives depending on disease manifestations.

Intra-articular corticosteroids given prior to antibiotic treatment have been implicated in a more chronic arthritis, but have also been associated with decreasing the duration of synovitis if given after the course of antibiotics [6].

9.9   Outcome

Lyme disease has an excellent prognosis [2, 4, 6, 7]. The vast majority of features are self-limited. Children with Lyme arthritis generally do very well with either the initial course of oral antibiotics or, if needed, an intravenous course (with or without an intra-articular injection of corticosteroids). If the arthritis does not resolve, then the diagnosis needs to be reconsidered. The anxiety surrounding the mythical "chronic Lyme disease" needs to be directly and compassionately dealt with early on to prevent unnecessary disability and prolonged courses of antibiotics [4, 7, 8].

TABLE 9.1 Treatment regimens for Lyme disease [5]

Agents (mg given per dose)

Doxycycline 100 mg PO twice daily (over age 8 years)

Amoxicillin 500 or 17 mg/kg PO three times daily (under age 9 years or pregnant)

Cefuroxime axetil 500 mg or 15 mg/kg PO twice daily

Erythromycin 500 mg or 12.5 mg/kg PO once daily (less effective)

Azithromycin 500 mg or 10 mg/kg PO (less effective)

Clarithromycin 500 mg or 7.5 mg/kg PO twice daily (less effective)

Penicillin G 4 million units or 50,000 units/kg IV every 4 h

Ceftriaxone sodium 2 g or 50–75 mg/kg IV single daily dose

Cefotaxime sodium 6 g or 50 mg/kg IV every 8 h

Erythema migrans

Doxycycline, amoxicillin, cefuroxime axetil, erythromycin, azithromycin or clarithromycin PO for 14–21 days (7 days for azithromycin)

Lyme arthritis

Doxycycline or amoxicillin PO for 21–28 days

If fails: ceftriaxone sodium or Penicillin G IV for 30 days

Bell palsy

Doxycycline or amoxicillin PO for 21–28 days

Central nervous system Lyme

Ceftriaxone sodium or penicillin G IV for 30 days

Alternatives: cefotaxime sodium or chloramphenicol IV for 30 days

Carditis

Mild: doxycycline or amoxicillin PO for 14–21 days

Severe: ceftriaxone sodium or penicillin G IV for 14–21 days

References

1. Steere AC, Malawista SE, Snydman DR, et al. Lyme arthritis: an epidemic of oligoarticular arthritis in children and adults in three Connecticut communities. Arthritis Rheum. 1977;20:7–17.
2. Sood SK. Lyme disease in children. Infect Dis Clin North Am. 2015;29:281–94.
3. Stanek G, Strle F. Lyme borreliosis. Lancet. 2003;362:1639–47.
4. Halperin JJ. Nervous system Lyme disease, chronic Lyme disease, and none of the above. Acta Neurol Belg. 2015;116:1–6.
5. Wormser GP, Dattwyler RJ, Shapiro ED, et al. The clinical assessment, treatment, and prevention of Lyme disease, human granulocytic anaplasmosis, and babesiosis: clinical practice guidelines by the Infectious Diseases Society of America. Clin Infect Dis. 2006;43:1089–134.
6. Bentas W, Karch H, Huppertz HI. Lyme arthritis in children and adolescents: outcome 12 months after initiation of antibiotic therapy. J Rheumatol. 2000;27:2025–30.
7. Oliveira CR, Shapiro ED. Update on persistent symptoms associated with Lyme disease. Curr Opin Pediatr. 2015;27:100–4.
8. Sigal LH, Patella SJ. Lyme arthritis as the incorrect diagnosis in pediatric and adolescent fibromyalgia. Pediatrics. 1992;90:523–8.

Chapter 10
Autoinflammatory Syndromes

10.1   Introduction and Approach

The most common cause of fever in childhood is infection. When the fever is prolonged or recurrent, the differential diagnosis widens to include unusual or occult infections, inflammatory and autoimmune diseases and malignancies. In the last two decades the autoinflammatory syndromes, a category of diseases often characterized by recurrent fever, were described. These are defined as recurrent attacks of inflammation, often multisystem, that are unprovoked (or triggered by a minor event) related to dysregulation of the innate immune system. Many of the syndromes are monogenic, and may be inherited in an autosomal dominant or recessive pattern. The inflammatory response is mediated primarily by interleukin (IL)-1 secreted by granulocytes and monocytes (Fig. 10.1). Unlike autoimmune diseases, there is a paucity of both autoantibodies and auto-reactive T cells [1]. Periodic/ recurrent fever syndromes were the former name for these diseases. However, fever is neither necessary nor recurrent in some of the syndromes. The spectrum of the autoinflammatory syndromes continues to expand in an exponential fashion and includes common diseases such as gout, type II diabetes and coronary artery disease [1]. This chapter is limited to describing the classic autoinflammatory syndromes, especially the monogenic diseases (Table 10.1). We refer

R.M. Laxer et al., *Pediatric Rheumatology in Clinical Practice*,   189
DOI 10.1007/978-3-319-13099-6_10,
© Springer-Verlag London 2016

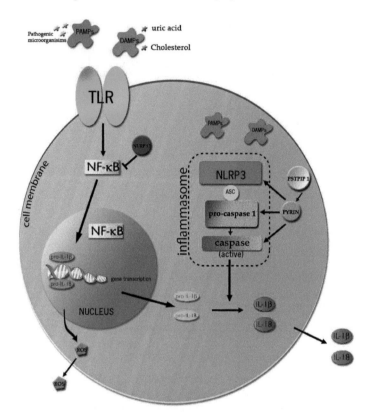

FIGURE 10.1 Schema of selected innate immune inflammatory pathways related to the autoinflammatory syndromes. The schema demonstrates the effect of external stimuli on the development of inflammation and the relationship of several regulatory proteins (pyrin, NLRP3, NLRP12, PSTPIP1) that when mutated result in the development of autoinflammatory diseases (Reprinted with permission from Hashkes [21]). *PAMP* pathogen associated molecular patterns, *DAMP* damage associated molecular patterns, *TLR* toll-like receptors, *NLR* nod-like receptors, *NLRPs* NLRs with pyrin-domain-containing-proteins, *IL* interleukin, *PSTPIP* proline-serine-threonine phosphatase-interacting protein, *ROS* reactive oxygen species, *NF-κB* nuclear factor kappa-light-chain-enhancer of activated B cells, *ASC* apoptosis-associated speck protein containing a caspase activation and recruitment domain

TABLE 10.1   The autoinflammatory syndromes

Familial Mediterranean Fever (FMF)

Mevalonate Kinase Deficiency (MKD) formerly Hyperimmunoglobulinemia D and Periodic Fever Syndrome (HIDS)

Tumor Necrosis Factor Receptor Associated Periodic Syndrome (TRAPS)

Cryopyrin Associated Periodic Syndromes (CAPS)

　Familial Cold Autoinflammatory Syndrome (FCAS)

　Muckle–Wells Syndrome (MWS)

　Neonatal Onset Multisystem Inflammatory Disease (NOMID) or Chronic Infantile Neurological Cutaneous and Articular Syndrome (CINCA)

Deficiencies in Receptor Antagonists

　Deficiency of the Interleukin (IL) 1 Receptor Antagonist (DIRA)

　Deficiency of the IL-36 Receptor Antagonist (DITRA)

Interferonopathies

　Nakajo-Nishimura Syndrome or Chronic Atypical Neutrophilic Dermatosis with Lipodystrophy and Elevated Temperature (CANDLE) Syndrome or Joint Contractures, Muscular Atrophy, Microcytic Anemia, and Panniculitis-Induced Lipodystrophy (JMP) Syndrome

　Stimulator of Interferon Genes (STING) Associated Vasculopathy with Onset in Infancy (SAVI)

Periodic Fever, Aphthous Stomatitis, Pharyngitis, and Adenitis Syndrome (PFAPA)

Chronic Recurrent Multifocal Osteomyelitis (CRMO)

Diseases discussed in this chapter; please refer to other references for a more comprehensive list and discussion of the autoinflammatory syndromes readers to other references that expand on rare autoinflammatory syndromes not described in this chapter [1]. Summaries of the clinical and genetic aspects of the major autoinflammatory syndromes described herein are in Tables 10.2 and 10.3.

Autoinflammatory diseases should be suspected in children (the onset can rarely occur in adulthood), with recurrent fever and increased acute phase reactants unexplained by infections and/or with episodic symptoms in various systems, especially the skin, gastrointestinal tract, chest, eyes, musculoskeletal and central nervous systems. A family history including features such as early-onset hearing loss, renal failure or amyloidosis may increase the suspicion of these diseases.

A complete history and physical examination are crucial and often the correct diagnosis can be reached even without obtaining genetic tests . Several pertinent questions can help characterize and differentiate between syndromes (Table 10.4) [1, 2]. It is important to examine patients during an attack, or if not possible, ask caregivers to carefully record attacks and take photos of significant physical findings. Laboratory markers of inflammation both during and between attacks should be obtained. In some syndromes attacks are only the "tip of the iceberg" and patients consistently have increased inflammatory indices, placing them at higher risk of developing amyloidosis. The major role of genetic testing is to confirm the clinical diagnosis and provide prognostic information [3]. Genetic testing needs interpretation by experienced practitioners, since there are many false positive ("polymorphisms") and negative results as well as variants of unknown significance.

10.2   Familial Mediterranean Fever (FMF)

FMF was the first recognized and is the most common monogenic autoinflammatory syndrome [1]. It is marked by serious morbidity and potential mortality if not treated adequately.

TABLE 10.2 Major clinical manifestations of the classic autoinflammatory syndromes

	FMF	MKD/HIDS	TRAPS	CAPS	PFAPA
Typical age of onset	80 % <10 years	<1 year	Any (25 % in adulthood)	Within first year	<5 years
Duration of attacks	0.5–3 days	3–7 days	>7 days	From 1 day to continuous[a]	3–7 days
Skin	Erysipelas-like	Various rashes	Painful migratory plaques	Urticaria	None
Musculoskeletal	Mono/ oligoarthritis	Arthralgia/ arthritis	Arthralgia/ myalgia	Arthralgia/arthritis[a]	None
	Myalgia			Irregular ossification[a]	
				Epiphyseal overgrowth[a]	

(continued)

TABLE 10.2 (continued)

	FMF	MKD/HIDS	TRAPS	CAPS	PFAPA
Abdominal/GI	Peritonitis Splenomegaly	Pain, diarrhea Splenomegaly	Pain, diarrhea Splenomegaly	Uncommon	Pain
Ocular	Rare	Conjunctivitis	Periorbital edema, conjunctivitis	Conjunctivitis to uveitis to papillitis/ papilledema[a]	None
Neurologic	Headaches	Rare	Rare	Headaches to sensorineural hearing loss to chronic meningitis[a]	Rare
Lymphadenopathy	None	Cervical to general	Uncommon	None	Cervical

Other features	Scrotal swelling	Vasculitis; aphthous		Frontal bossing	Tonsillitis; aphthous
Amyloidosis	Yes	Rare	Yes	Yes[a]	None
Treatment	Colchicine, anti IL-1	Anti IL-1, etanercept	Anti IL-1, etanercept	Anti IL-1	Corticosteroids[b] T&A

FMF familial Mediterranean fever, *MKD/HIDS* mevalonate kinase deficiency/hyperimmunoglobulinemia D syndrome, *TRAPS* tumor necrosis factor receptor associated periodic syndrome, *CAPS* cryopyrin associated periodic syndrome, *PFAPA* periodic fever, aphthous stomatitis, pharyngitis, adenitis syndrome, *IL* interleukin, *T&A* tonsillectomy ± adenoidectomy

[a] Depends on CAPS subtype

[b] One dose given at start of attack

TABLE 10.3 Genetics of the classic autoinflammatory syndromes

	FMF	MKD/HIDS	TRAPS	CAPS	PFAPA
Inheritance	AR, occasional AD	AR	AD	AD	Unknown, frequent family history
Chromosome	16p13	12q24	12p13	1q44	Unknown
Gene	*MEFV*	*MVK*	*TNFRSF1A*	*NLRP3*	Unknown
Protein	Pyrin (Marenostrin)	Mevalonate kinase	Tumor necrosis factor receptor 1	Cryopyrin	Unknown

AR autosomal recessive, *AD* autosomal dominant, *FMF* familial Mediterranean fever, *MKD/HIDS* mevalonate kinase deficiency/hyperimmunoglobulinemia D syndrome, *TRAPS* tumor necrosis factor receptor associated periodic syndrome, *CAPS* cryopyrin associated periodic syndrome *PFAPA* periodic fever, aphthous stomatitis, pharyngitis, adenitis syndrome

TABLE 10.4 Important history items in investigating autoinflammatory syndromes

Age of onset
Ethnicity (e.g. Mediterranean, Netherlands)
Consanguinity and family history
Attack triggers (e.g. cold, vaccines, stress, exercise)
Duration of attacks
Disease-free intervals between attacks (including periodicity)
Clinical manifestations (e.g. fever, skin, gastrointestinal, chest, musculoskeletal, eye, neurologic)
Response to therapy (colchicine, corticosteroids, TNF and IL-1 inhibitors)

TNF tumor necrosis factor, *IL* interleukin

10.2.1   Etiology

FMF is due to a mutation in the *MEFV* gene, located on the short arm of chromosome 16, that codes for a protein called "pyrin" or "Marenostrin" [1]. This gene is expressed primarily in granulocytes. There is debate on the role of the protein in the regulation (augmentation or reduction) of inflammation via the pyrin and NLRP3 inflammasomes and IL-1 activation (Fig. 10.1). There are other membrane and intracellular signals that are crucial for activation of the pyrin protein. At least 250 distinct mutations in *MEFV* have been identified with only about 50 %, mainly on exon 10, causing disease. Some mutations, particularly the common methionine for valine substitution at position 694 (M694V), and methionine for isoleucine at positions 694 and 680 (M694I and M680I) mutations seem to correlate with the disease severity and outcome. While generally considered to be an autosomal recessive disease, about 30 % of the patients have only one identified (heterozygous) mutation, thus FMF is not exclusively an autosomal recessive disease.

10.2.2   Epidemiology

FMF affects mainly populations of Mediterranean origin, especially Sephardic Jews, Armenians, Turks and Arabs. Nearly 80 % of patients experience their first attack before the age of 10 years, and 90 % before 20 years.

10.2.3   Clinical Features

FMF is characterized by attacks lasting between 12 and 72 h, which include the abrupt onset of fever accompanied by serosal inflammation. Peritonitis, seen in ~90 % of patients, may mimic an acute surgical abdomen. Constipation is more common than diarrhea. Pleuritis occurs in 30–45 %. Arthritis occurs in 25–75 % of patients, (dependent on series and geography of patients) commonly presenting as an acute large joint mono- or oligoarthritis. Five to 10 % of patients develop a chronic destructive arthritis of the hips and sacroiliac joints. Erysipelas-like skin lesions, primarily on the lower extremities, can accompany attacks (~25 %; Fig. 10.2). In younger children fever may be the only symptom. Other manifestations include exercise-induced (leg) myalgia, orchitis, headaches (representing aseptic meningitis) splenomegaly, growth delay and short stature. There is a higher prevalence of vasculitis including leukocytoclastic vasculitis, polyarteritis nodosa (PAN) and prolonged febrile myalgia in patients with FMF. Intervals between attacks vary from several days to months and may be triggered by stress, exercise, menstrual periods, infection and trauma. Patients are well between attacks, but may have elevated inflammatory markers. Untreated male patients living in the Middle East, with "severe" mutations (e.g. M694V) and a family history are at an increased risk to develop amyloidosis. Amyloidosis usually presents with proteinuria.

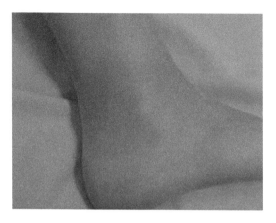

FIGURE 10.2 Erysipelas-like erythema overlying the right lateral malleolus in a 14-year-old girl with familial Mediterranean fever (FMF) (Courtesy of Dr. Shai Padeh, Sheba Medical Center, Israel)

10.2.4   Laboratory Features and Diagnosis

The diagnosis of FMF should be made clinically based on the characteristic clinical manifestations, response to treatment with colchicine and family history. Diagnostic criteria for adults and children have been validated [3]. Genetic testing is not diagnostic since as many as 30 % of patients do not have mutations on both copies of the *MEFV* gene. Acute phase reactants are increased during attacks and in some patients remain elevated even between attacks. Elevated fibrinogen levels are not specific to FMF. It is important to perform urinalysis at regular intervals to monitor for proteinuria which may be the first evidence of amyloidosis.

10.2.5   Treatment

Colchicine is the treatment of choice [4, 5]. It reduces the frequency and severity of attacks in the vast majority of patients and prevents the development of amyloidosis, even in poor responders. A partial response in seen in ~30–40 % of patients and ~5 % are non-responders. NSAIDs are effective in the treatment of arthritis. IV fluids and analgesics may be helpful in peritoneal attacks. Since it is not possible to predict who will develop amyloidosis, colchicine use should be life-long, even in the absence of symptoms. The dose of colchicine used is 0.5–3 mg per day (dependent on weight/age/response) [4]. In high doses colchicine is more effective in divided doses with less adverse effects but adherence may be affected. The major side effects are abdominal pain and diarrhea, often related to secondary lactose intolerance. Periodic monitoring of CBC, liver and renal function is necessary. Long-term colchicine use is safe, including during pregnancy [1, 4, 5]. IL-1 inhibition is highly effective in most patients non-responsive or intolerant to colchicine [4, 6].

10.2.6   Outcome

The use of colchicine has dramatically improved the outcome of patients with FMF, 50 % of whom eventually developed amyloidosis without treatment.

10.3   Mevalonate Kinase Deficiency (MKD)

Mevalonate kinase deficiency (MKD), previously called hyperimmunoglobulinemia D syndrome with periodic fever (HIDS), was first described in a group of Dutch patients in 1984 [7]. MKD is a monogenic metabolic disease marked by recurrent attacks of fever and systemic inflammation, beginning very early in life, in association with elevated levels of serum IgD in many but not all patients (see below).

10.3.1   Etiology

MKD is an autosomal recessive disease. Mutations of the mevalonate kinase (*MVK*) gene, located on the long arm of chromosome 12, result in reduced activity of the enzyme catalyzing the metabolism of mevalonate in the isoprenoid and cholesterol biosynthesis pathway. Severe reductions in enzyme activity (<1 % activity) result in the disease mevalonic aciduria, primarily a neurologic disease. In MKD there is usually between 5 % and 15 % enzyme activity. How the metabolic defect leads to bouts of severe repeated inflammation is not fully understood and may be related to deficiency in geranylgeranyl and other isoprenoid substrates that regulate inflammatory pathways.

10.3.2   Epidemiology

MKD usually starts within the first year of life. Many of the affected patients described are of Dutch or Western European origin.

10.3.3   Clinical Features

The attacks of fever are longer compared to FMF, lasting 3–7 days, with an irregular periodicity, anywhere from once every 2 weeks to every several months. Fever rises abruptly, often with chills and climbs quickly up to 40 °C (104 °F). Usually, there is no precipitant, but trauma, infection, and, in particular, immunizations may initiate an attack. Prominent symptoms during attacks are gastrointestinal (nausea, vomiting, diarrhea, abdominal pain). Other frequent symptoms are arthralgia/arthritis, tender cervical lymphadenopathy and oral aphthous ulcers. Splenomegaly and hepatomegaly are common in children, but rare in adults. A variety of rashes, including macular, papular, mobilliform, urticarial, nodular, purpuric, and erythema multiforme/nodosum/marginatum, on the trunk, limbs, and palms are frequent during attacks (Fig. 10.3). Attacks tend to lessen in frequency with age. Amyloidosis is rare (<3 %) [8].

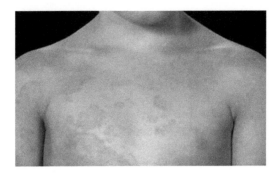

FIGURE 10.3 The rash of mevalonate kinase deficiency (MKD) is typically over the whole body, including the palms of the hand. It is a polymorphic rash and can be mobilliform or can appear, as in this figure, like erythema marginatum

10.3.4   Laboratory Features and Diagnosis

The typical clinical pattern, together with a raised serum IgD, increased urinary mevalonic acid (mainly during a febrile attack) and the presence of *MVK* mutations provide the diagnosis. However, some classic, especially younger, patients have normal IgD levels and elevated IgD levels may be found in patients with other autoinflammatory syndromes. Elevated levels of serum IgA often accompany the high IgD levels. Elevated acute phase reactants are seen during attacks. Most patients have homozygous or compound heterozygous mutations in the *MVK* gene, with V377I being the most common.

10.3.5   Treatment

Mild attacks may respond to NSAIDs and corticosteroids. Colchicine and statins are not effective. In patients who have frequent and/or severe attacks IL-1 inhibition (anakinra and canakinumab) are effective in about 50–60 % of cases and TNF inhibition with etanercept in about 40 %, although complete response may be more common with use of IL-1 inhibitors [6, 8].

10.3.6   Outcome

The frequency and severity of attacks lessen with age [8]. Fortunately, long-term sequelae, like amyloidosis and mortality, are rare (~3 %). The development of renal angiomyolipoma has been reported in some patients.

10.4   Tumor Necrosis Factor-Receptor-Associated Periodic Syndrome (TRAPS)

TRAPS was originally described in a large Irish/Scottish family cohort and so was called familial Hibernian fever. The genetic cause of TRAPS, the most common autosomal dominant autoinflammatory disease, was discovered in 1999, soon after the discovery of the genetic cause of FMF [1, 9].

10.4.1   Etiology

TRAPS is due to a mutation of the *TNFRSF1A* gene on the short arm of chromosome 12, responsible for coding the type I TNF p55 receptor. The most significant mutations alter the structure of the two extracellular domains of the TNF receptor, through disruption of cysteine disulfide bonds. It is clear the pathogenesis of TRAPS is more complicated than the initial hypothesis of a decrease in the shedding of mutated membrane bound TNF receptors leading to an increase of unopposed serum TNF. Other hypotheses includes defects in intracellular trafficking of the receptor leading to deficiencies in TNF induced apoptosis and stimulation of intracellular inflammation via reactive oxygen species [1, 9].

10.4.2   Epidemiology

TRAPS is an autosomal dominant disorder, but sporadic cases do occur. It has been reported most frequently in families with Celtic origins in Ireland and Scotland, but the disease is worldwide, including in Africa. Most patients have their onset in childhood, but symptoms may be delayed in ~25 % until adulthood.

10.4.3   Clinical Features

Usually, there is no precipitant, but minor trauma, stress, infection, and, in particular vigorous exercise may trigger an attack. Attacks typically are much longer in duration compared to MKD or FMF, lasting between 1 and 3 weeks, although, they may be shorter in patients with non-cysteine mutations. A characteristic painful, migrating erythematosus (macular and/or plaque) rash which represents fasciitis is a unique feature of TRAPS (Fig. 10.4). Rashes are often accompanied by myalgias, which are also often migratory. Ocular features, particularly periorbital edema also help differentiate TRAPS from other autoinflammatory syndromes. Conjunctivitis is common. Other clinical features include fever, colicky abdominal pain, diarrhea or constipation, arthralgia of large joints (rarely arthritis), testicular pain, pleuritic and pericardial chest pain and oral ulcers. Amyloidosis may develop in up to 25 % of patients [10].

10.4.4   Laboratory Features and Diagnosis

Acute phase reactants are elevated during and often also between attacks. It is important to perform urinalysis at regular intervals to monitor for proteinuria and amyloidosis. Identification of mutations in the *TNFRSF1A* gene is necessary to confirm a diagnosis of TRAPS.

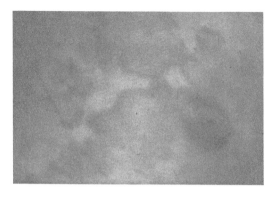

FIGURE 10.4 This rash was from a boy with tumor necrosis factor receptor associated periodic syndrome (TRAPS). It is a painful erythematosus rash that migrates from the trunk to the limbs

10.4.5   Treatment

Attacks may be ameliorated by NSAIDs but usually corticosteroids are needed, in increasing doses over time. Therefore, alternative treatments are necessary. Soluble TNF receptor, subcutaneous etanercept, given twice or three times per week may be beneficial, but often acute phase reactants remain elevated and the effect wears off with time. Treatment with monoclonal anti-TNF antibodies may worsen disease. IL-1 inhibition appears to be the most effective therapy [6]. Several case reports of treatment with IL-6 inhibition (tocilizumab) have been reported.

10.4.6   Outcome

Attacks, although irregular, are life-long. Amyloidosis develops in approximately 25 % of patients not treated with biologic therapy.

10.5   The Cryopyrin Associated Periodic Syndromes (CAPS)

The following three syndromes are all characterized by auto-somal dominant transmission (although sporadic cases do occur), early age of onset and mutations in the *NLRP3* gene (previously called *NALP3*, *CIAS1* and *PYPAF1*) [11]. This gene is located on chromosome 1 and encodes a protein called cryopyrin. Cryopyrin, like pyrin, is expressed in granu-locytes as well as monocytes and chondrocytes. Some muta-tions are associated with a specific phenotype while others can overlap between the various phenotypes, suggesting that other factors play a role in determining the phenotypic expression of the mutation [11]. Cryopyrin is an important protein in the NLRP3 inflammasome responsible for activat-ing caspase 1 (Fig. 10.1). Caspase 1 cleaves pro-interleukin (IL)-1β to the active IL-1β. *NLRP3* mutations result in a gain of function of cryopyrin and the inflammasome resulting in increased production of IL-1β and inflammation even in the absence of an external stimulation by bacteria, viruses or other environmental triggers. All of the CAPS phenotypes are highly responsive to IL-1 inhibition, which is the treat-ment of choice. Early diagnosis and treatment are necessary to prevent complications and damage, which is usually irreversible.

10.5.1   Familial Cold Autoinflammatory Syndrome (FCAS)

FCAS usually begins very early in infancy and is transmitted in an autosomal dominant pattern with complete penetrance. Attacks are precipitated 2–3 h after general cold exposure (including air-conditioning) and consist of low-grade fever, chills, sweating, extreme thirst, fatigue, non-pruritic urticarial-like rash, arthralgia, myalgia conjunctivitis and headaches. Attacks, which can be disabling, peak 6–8 h after exposure and last up to 24 h. Acute phase reactants are elevated during attacks. While attacks occur throughout life, amyloidosis is rare.

10.5.2 Muckle–Wells Syndrome (MWS)

MWS is characterized by autosomal dominant transmission, early age of onset (although can present in later childhood) and unpredictable attacks, lasting 1–3 days. While it has many similarities to FCAS, attacks generally occur spontaneously and are more severe than in FCAS. In addition to FCAS attacks may include arthritis, uveitis, more severe headaches and even aseptic meningitis. Patients may have clubbing. Complications include amyloidosis (~25 %) and sensorineural deafness, usually starting in adolescence with hearing loss of high frequency sounds. While highly effective in preventing attacks, IL-1 inhibition reverses established hearing loss in only 20–33 % of patients.

10.5.3 Neonatal Onset Multisystem Inflammatory Disease (NOMID)

NOMID, also known in Europe as the chronic infantile neurological cutaneous and articular (CINCA) syndrome, is the most severe form of CAPS starting very early in infancy. The disease is persistent, not episodic, with the typical non-pruritic urticarial-like rash often present at birth (Fig. 10.5). In addition to features seen in MWS, patients have chronic meningitis manifesting with headache, irritability and vomiting, with increased opening pressure and pleocytosis, often leading to hydrocephalus, developmental and intellectual delays and disabilities. Papillitis and papilledema are common and can lead to blindness. By 2 years of age about 50 % of NOMID patients develop an arthropathy marked by distinctive radiographic epiphyseal and/or metaphyseal abnormalities with prema-

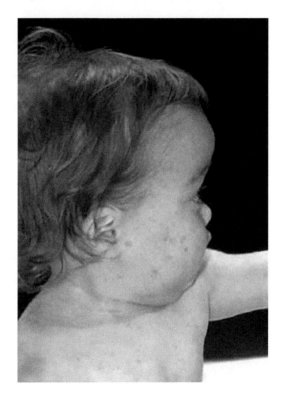

FIGURE 10.5 This patient with neonatal onset multisystem inflammatory disease (NOMID)/chronic infantile neurological cutaneous and articular syndrome (CINCA) shows the typical frontal bossing and the urticarial-like rash on the face

ture and irregular ossification and bony overgrowth. These radiographic changes are dramatic and affect mainly the knees, ankles, wrists and elbows. Patients have characteristic morphologic features of frontal bossing (Fig. 10.5), saddle nose, macrocephaly, clubbing, wrinkled skin and short stature. Prior to the discovery of the effectiveness of IL-1 inhibitors 20 % of NOMID patients died by age 20 years and many others developed amyloidosis. While generally effective, IL-1 inhibitors are not effective in treating the arthropathy of NOMID. Higher doses of IL-1 inhibitors are needed to treat NOMID compared to FCAS and MWS and often there is not complete control of headaches and increased intracranial pressure, perhaps due to inadequate penetration of drug through the blood brain barrier [11].

10.6   Deficiencies in Cytokine Receptor Antagonists

Some of the receptor antagonists function as natural protein inhibitors of inflammatory processes by competing with pro-inflammatory cytokines for membrane or intracellular receptors. At least two autoinflammatory syndromes have been described related to mutations in genes that encode receptor antagonists.

10.6.1   Deficiency of the IL-1 Receptor Antagnonist (DIRA)

DIRA is an autosomal recessive disease described in families from Newfoundland, Puerto Rico, Lebanon and Southern Netherlands which is caused by a mutation (or deletion) in the *IL1RN* gene on the long-arm of chromosome 2, which encodes the IL-1 receptor antagonist [12].

DIRA presents at birth or shortly after with a sterile pustular rash, multifocal osteomyelitis with lytic bone lesions, nail pits, oral ulcers and respiratory distress with pneumonitis. Treatment with anakinra, an IL-1 receptor antagonist, is remarkably effcctive and prevents the morbidity and mortality of DIRA. Prior to the discovery of effective treatment patients developed severe skeletal deformities, failure to thrive and often succumbed to the disease.

10.6.2   Deficiency of the IL-36 Receptor Antagonist (DITRA)

DITRA is a rare autosomal receive disease described in Tunisian and several European families. DITRA is caused by a mutation in the *IL36RN* gene at the long arm of chromosome 3, near the *IL1RN* gene, that encodes the IL-36 receptor antagonist [13].

DITRA can start from infancy to mid-adulthood and pregnancy has been a trigger in several patients. Patients develop flares of high fever lasting 1–3 days and a generalized pustular rash lasting days to weeks. About 30 % develop arthritis and a chronic course of psoriasis vulgaris. Treatment includes use of oral retinoids, immunosuppressive medications; successful treatment with IL-1 and TNF inhibitors has been reported. There is a high mortality rate from sepsis related from the loss of the skin barrier during acute attacks.

10.7   Interferonopathies

These diseases relate to uncontrolled up regulation of type I interferon signaling and gene expression (mainly α and β) causing autoinflammation [14]. Recently two monogenic diseases have been described. These diseases are not responsive to conventional anti-inflammatory therapies, including IL-1 inhibition, but may respond to inhibition of the interferon signaling pathways by Janus kinase inhibitors.

10.7.1   Proteosome Associated Autoinflammatory Syndrome

Proteosomes are large intracellular complexes that degrade unnecessary or abnormal proteins. The *PSMB8* gene located on the short arm of chromosome 6 encodes a ring subunit in the proteosome. Mutations in that gene cause an autosomal recessive autoinflammatory disease related to cellular stress leading to stimulation of the Type I and II interferon pathways [15]. Three conditions that probably represent one disorder have been described. The Nakajo-Nishimura syndrome was described in Japan; the joint contractures, muscular atrophy, microcytic anemia, and panniculitis-induced lipodystrophy (JMP) syndrome in Spain, and elsewhere the chronic atypical neutrophilic dermatosis with lipodystrophy and elevated temperature (CANDLE) syndrome. These syndromes are characterized by early onset (usually in the first year of life) recurrent fevers, purpuric rash and erythematous/violaceous plaques representing panniculitis primarily on the upper limbs, face and eyelids, progressive lipodystrophy, arthralgia/arthritis and joint deformities, hepatomegaly, failure to thrive with anemia and increased acute phase reactants. Patients may also develop hypertrichosis, acanthosis nigricans, alopecia areata, scleritis, interstitial lung disease and aseptic meningitis.

10.7.2 Stimulator of Interferon Genes (STING) Associated Vasculopathy with Onset in Infancy (SAVI)

This rare autosomal dominant disease results from gain of function de-novo mutations in the *TMEM173* gene, encoding STING, located on the long-arm of chromosome 5 [16]. In the first weeks of life patients develop a systemic inflammatory disease with capillary vasculopathy/vasculitis characterized by a violaceous pustular scaly rash on the digits, nose, cheeks and ears with telangiectasia that may progress to acral necrosis and gangrene. The rash worsens with cold exposure. Most patients develop interstitial lung disease and have episodes of low grade fever and failure to thrive. Acute phase reactants are markedly elevated. Most patients succumb to pulmonary disease or infection.

10.8   Periodic Fever, Aphthous Stomatitis, Pharyngitis, and Adenitis (PFAPA) Syndrome

PFAPA syndrome is probably the most common autoinflammatory fever syndrome worldwide. Attacks start in early life, usually between 1.5 and 5 years of age. It is characterized by periodic attacks occurring every 2–8 weeks, with parents often able to predict when attacks will occur [2]. Attacks, which typically last between 3 and 7 days, consist of abrupt fever spikes, tonsillitis/pharyngitis (no pathogens identified) and tender cervical lymphadenopathy. Painful oral ulcers are common during attacks. Not all features develop consistently with each attack. Some patients develop abdominal pain, arthralgia/myalgia and headaches. Patients are completely well between attacks (including laboratory markers of inflammation) [17]. Although no genetic cause has been identified, there is often a family history of PFAPA or of a tonsillectomy (suggesting treatment for this disease). Many patients in the Middle East carry a heterozygous mutation on the *MEFV* gene. Investigation for other autoinflammatory disorders, particularly TRAPS, MKD and cyclic neutropenia is necessary in patients with atypical features. Corticosteroids given at the onset of attacks (between 0.6 and 2 mg/kg of prednisone or prednisolone) are very effective in aborting attacks. However, in 33–50 % of patients attacks may become more frequent. Prophylactic medical treatment, including colchicine and cimetidine, are effective in preventing attacks in only 30–50 % of patients (colchicine is likely more effective). Tonsillectomy (±adenoidectomy) is curative in >85 % of properly diagnosed patients [18]. The outcome is good and most (but not all) patients generally "outgrow" the disease during their second decade.

10.9 Chronic Recurrent Multifocal Osteomyelitis (CRMO)

CRMO is a non-infectious autoinflammatory bone disease. It is more common in females (2:1) and the most common onset is during early adolescence, It is usually sporadic, however, up to 25 % of patients have a positive family history, mainly for psoriasis or inflammatory bowel disease. The etiology is usually unknown, however, there are several rare genetic autoinflammatory bone disorders resembling CRMO including DIRA (described above), Majeed syndrome (CRMO with congenital dyserythropoietic anemia) and cherubism (bone degradation of the jaws) [19]. CRMO can be associated with various systemic disease, like Behcet disease and Takayasu arteritis in addition to psoriasis and inflammatory bowel disease.

Patients develop episodes of bone pain with or without low-grade fever with spontaneous remissions (including radiologic) and relapses. Radiographs show osteolytic lesions surrounded by sclerotic bone and often periostitis. Most commonly, lesions are found in the metaphysis of long bones. There is also frequent involvement of the clavicle, ribs, mandible, pelvis and vertebral bodies. Asymptomatic lesions are often detected by technetium nuclear bone scans or whole-body MRI scans; the latter is the preferred form of radiographic investigation. Associated features are common and include palmoplantar pustulosis, psoriasis, pyoderma gangrenosum, arthritis, sacroiliitis, inflammatory bowel disease and features of the SAPHO syndrome (synovitis, acne, pustulosis, hyperostosis and osteitis) [20]. Sequelae may develop in nearly 50 % of patients with bone sequelae resulting in leg length inequality and disability, occurring more often in males.

First line therapy consists of NSAIDs with occasional need for corticosteroids. Methotrexate and sulfasalazine are occasionally used as second line medications. In more severe cases (including vertebral involvement) bisphospho-nates and TNF inhibitors have been used with a generally good effect. The role of IL-1 inhibitors is still under investigation.

10.10   The Outcome of Patients with Undiagnosed Non-infectious Recurrent Fever

Despite the major advances in the autoinflammatory syndromes in the last decade more than 60 % of children with recurrent fever still go undiagnosed at tertiary centers. The majority of these children do well with resolution of their febrile episodes or decrease in the frequency and severity. Only a small minority will later develop a recognizable auto-inflammatory or rheumatic disease.

10.11   Summary

- Autoinflammatory syndromes should be suspected in young children with recurrent fevers without an infectious source as well as in patients with recurrent symptoms in other systems particularly the skin, gastrointestinal and musculoskeletal systems.
- Family history is extremely helpful in making the diagnosis, but the disease may also be sporadic as the result of a spontaneous mutation.
- A careful history and documentations of attacks, including photographs of pertinent findings, are crucial in diagnosing and differentiating between autoinflammatory syndromes.
- Genetic testing is available for many of the autoinflammatory syndromes but the diagnosis is still clinically based for the majority of the syndromes. Genetic testing has a primarily confirmatory and prognostic role; the results should be interpreted by experts in these syndromes.

- Treatment is usually effective and based on the underlying molecular defect.
- Early treatment may prevent long-term morbidity and even mortality.

References

1. Hashkes PJ, Toker O. Autoinflammatory syndromes. Pediatr Clin North Am. 2012;59:447–70.
2. Federici S, Gattorno M. A practical approach to the diagnosis of autoinflammatory diseases in childhood. Best Pract Res Clin Rheumatol. 2014;28:263–76.
3. Federici S, Sormani MP, Ozen S, et al. for the Paediatric Rheumatology International Trials Organisation (PRINTO) and Eurofever Project. Evidence-based provisional clinical classification criteria for autoinflammatory periodic fevers. Ann Rheum Dis. 2015;74:799–805.
4. Hentgen V, Grateau G, Kone-Paut I, et al. Evidence-based recommendations for the practical management of familial Mediterranean fever. Semin Arthritis Rheum. 2013;43:387–91.
5. Padeh S, Gerstein M, Berkun Y. Colchicine is a safe drug in children with familial Mediterranean fever. J Pediatr. 2012;161:1142–6.
6. Ter Haar N, Lachmann H, Ozen S, et al. for the Paediatric Rheumatology International Trials Organisation (PRINTO) and the Eurofever/Eurotraps Projects. Treatment of autoinflammatory diseases: results from the Eurofever Registry and a literature review. Ann Rheum Dis. 2013;72:678–85.
7. Drenth JP, Haagsma CJ, van der Meer JW. Hyperimmunoglobulinemia D and periodic fever syndrome. The clinical spectrum in a series of 50 patients. Medicine (Baltimore). 1994;73:133–44.
8. van der Hilst JC, Bodar EJ, Barron KS, et al. International HIDS study group. Long-term follow-up, clinical features, and quality of life in a series of 103 patients with hyperimmunoglobulinemia D syndrome. Medicine (Baltimore). 2008;87:301–10.
9. Lachmann HJ, Papa R, Gerhold K, et al. for the Paediatric Rheumatology International Trials Organisation (PRINTO), the EUROTRAPS and the Eurofever Project. The phenotype of TNF receptor-associated autoinflammatory syndrome (TRAPS)

at presentation: a series of 158 cases from the Eurofever/ EUROTRAPS international registry. Ann Rheum Dis. 2014;73:2160–7.

10. Cantarini L, Lucherini OM, Muscari I, et al. Tumour necrosis factor receptor-associated periodic syndrome (TRAPS): state of the art and future perspectives. Autoimmun Rev. 2012;12:38–43.

11. Hashkes PJ, Laxer RM. The Cryopyrin-associated periodic syndromes: CAPS is underrecognized, undiagnosed and undertreated. Rheumatologist. 2014;9:18–22.

12. Aksentijevich I, Masters SL, Ferguson PJ, et al. An autoinflammatory disease with deficiency of the interleukin-1-receptor antagonist. N Engl J Med. 2009;360:2426–37.

13. Marrakchi S, Guigue P, Renshaw BR, et al. Interleukin-36-receptor antagonist deficiency and generalized pustular psoriasis. N Engl J Med. 2011;365:620–8.

14. Crow YJ. Type I interferonopathies: mendelian type I interferon up-regulation. Curr Opin Immunol. 2015;32:7–12.

15. McDermott A, Jacks J, Kessler M, Emanuel PD, Gao L. Proteasome-associated autoinflammatory syndromes: advances in pathogeneses, clinical presentations, diagnosis, and management. Int J Dermatol. 2015;54:121–9.

16. Liu Y, Jesus AA, Marrero B, et al. Activated STING in a vascular and pulmonary syndrome. N Engl J Med. 2014;371:507–18.

17. Hofer M, Pillet P, Cochard MM, et al. International periodic fever, aphthous stomatitis, pharyngitis, cervical adenitis syndrome cohort: description of distinct phenotypes in 301 patients. Rheumatology (Oxford). 2014;53:1125–9.

18. Burton MJ, Pollard AJ, Ramsden JD, Chong LY, Venekamp RP. Tonsillectomy for periodic fever, aphthous stomatitis, pharyngitis and cervical adenitis syndrome (PFAPA). Cochrane Database Syst Rev. 2014;9:CD008669.

19. Hedrich CM, Hofmann SR, Pablik J, Morbach H, Girschick HJ. Autoinflammatory bone disorders with special focus on chronic recurrent multifocal osteomyelitis (CRMO). Pediatr Rheumatol Online J. 2013;11:47.

20. Wipff J, Costantino F, Lemelle I, et al. A large national cohort of French patients with chronic recurrent multifocal osteitis. Arthritis Rheumatol. 2015;67:1128–37.

21. Hashkes PJ, Toker O. Autoinflammatory syndromes. Pediatr Clin North Am. 2012;59:455.

Chapter 11
Acute Rheumatic Fever and Post-Streptococcal Arthritis

11.1   Introduction

Acute rheumatic fever (ARF) is one of the first rheumatic diseases to be described centuries ago. It is one of the unique rheumatic diseases that is causally related to a preceding infection, i.e. pharyngitis caused by Group A β hemolytic Streptococci. Post-streptococcal arthritis (PSRA) has more recently been defined. Neither follows streptococcal infection of the skin, which can, however, cause an immune complex mediated glomerulonephritis.

11.2   Acute Rheumatic Fever

11.2.1   Definition

In 1944, Jones established criteria for diagnosing ARF that has undergone several revisions. The 1992 criteria are shown in Table 11.1 [1].

R.M. Laxer et al., *Pediatric Rheumatology in Clinical Practice*,   217
DOI 10.1007/978-3-319-13099-6_11,
© Springer-Verlag London 2016

TABLE 11.1 Jones criteria to establish the diagnosis of acute rheumatic fever (ARF): requires 2 of the major criteria or 1 major and 2 minor criteria

Major (% typically affected)	Minor
Carditis (50–70 %)	Prolonged PR interval
Arthritis (migratory) (70 %)	Arthralgia (cannot use if also has arthritis)
Erythema marginatum (<5 %)	
Nodules (subcutaneous) (<5 %)	Increased ESR or CRP
Chorea (15 %)	Fever

Also requires supporting evidence of antecedent group A streptococcal infection by throat culture, rapid streptococcal antigen test or elevated/rising streptococcal antibody titers (anti-streptolysin-O, anti-deoxyribonuclease B)

ESR erythrocyte sedimentation rate, *CRP* C-reactive protein

11.2.2   Epidemiology

The incidence in developed countries is probably <1 per 100,000 and in developing countries (and certain at risk populations) over 100 per 100,000. It is more common in Pacific islanders (Mauri, Samoa), Australian aborigines, in South America, the Indian subcontinent and the Middle East. Localized outbreaks are not unusual in developed countries. It most typically affects children aged 5–15 years old, and is rare under the age of 4 years [2, 3].

11.2.3   Etiology

The inciting agent is Group A β hemolytic *Streptococcal* pharyngitis in a susceptible host. Streptococci M protein and hyaluronate cross react (molecular mimicry) with human myocardium, myosin, brain, cartilage, and synovium [4]. There are about 85 M serotypes, but only several are rheumatogenic, particularly M3 and 18. A thick polysaccharide capsule may render the streptococcus more rheumatogenic. The host factors may include having HLA DRB1*16, DR2 among blacks and DR4 among Caucasians and a B-cell lymphocyte cell surface marker known as D8/17. The latter has been reported in >90 % of children with ARF and only 14 % of controls [5].

11.2.4 Clinical Manifestations

Arthritis affects about 70 % of children with ARF (Table 11.1). The arthritis is typically migratory, lasting hours to a few days in any given joint, with large joints (but not only) preferentially involved. It is associated with extreme pain (out of proportion to the degree of swelling) and even redness that responds rapidly to aspirin or other nonsteroidal anti-inflammatory drugs (NSAIDs). The carditis is described as a pancarditis and is present is 50–70 % of cases (more in endemic areas). However, the most common and important cardiac manifestation is endocarditis with involvement of the mitral more than the aortic valve, but only rarely the tricuspid and pulmonary valves. Myocarditis with congestive heart failure can occur early and is manifest in about 5 % of children with ARF. Mild pericarditis is often seen. Young children may present with heart failure and only minimal arthritis or fever [3]. Erythema marginatum is manifest early on as a serpiginous, nonpruritic erythematous rash, usually centrally located and migratory (Fig. 11.1). Two to 3 weeks later, painless subcutaneous nodules on the extensor surfaces (hands, feet, back and occiput) may develop and last about 3 weeks; they are associated with severe carditis. The last major manifestation to arise, 2–6 months later, is chorea (St. Vitus' dance) and may be the only evidence of ARF. It is much more common in girls, and is manifest by choreiform movements of the arms, face and tongue. A rhythmic hand

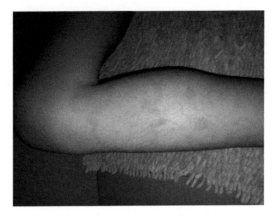

FIGURE 11.1 Erythema marginatum in a patient with acute rheumatic fever

squeezing (milk maid grip) and pronator sign of outstretched arms are typical physical findings. Patients develop handwriting changes, emotional lability and obsessive-compulsive behaviors. Chorea is worse with anxiety/stress and resolves during sleep. The movements last 6 weeks to 6 months [6]. Early in the course of ARF the minor manifestations are present, including a remittent fever, generally over 39 °C (102 °F) and arthralgia. Although not part of the criteria, abdominal pain responsive to NSAIDs and epistaxis can occur.

11.2.5   Laboratory Features

It is imperative to establish a prior streptococcal infection as often there is no history of a recent prior infection. A throat culture is positive in 20 % of cases. The antistreptolysin O (ASO) titre is elevated in only 80 % of children with ARF. Adding a second test, generally the anti-deoxyribonuclease B (anti-DNase B) will capture over 95 % of children with prior streptococcal infections. The strepto-zyme test is not sensitive or specific enough to be routinely used to establish, by itself, either ARF or PSRA. Other streptococcal antigens are not routinely tested for in most hospitals (including antihyaluronidase). Antibodies should rise at least fourfold between acute and convalescent sera, but the criteria state only a twofold increase or fall is sufficient if the initial values are not convincing of a prior streptococcal infection.

11.2.6   Establishing the Diagnosis

The diagnosis requires evidence of prior streptococcal infection and two major or one major and two minor criteria. Exceptions are chorea, the presence of rheumatic heart disease, and an illness like ARF in someone who has already suffered rheumatic heart damage so the presence of active carditis is not certain [1].

11.2.7   Treatment

Children with ARF should be treated initially for streptococcus and then prophylactic antibiotics should be given according to Table 11.2 [7]. Some studies suggest high-risk patients should have parental prophylaxis every 3 weeks rather than every 4 weeks, particularly in endemic regions. The duration of prophylaxis is dictated by the valvular disease. In patient without (or with resolved) carditis prophylaxis should last 5 years or up to 21 years of age (whichever is later). Current recommendations are for indefinite prophylaxis in patients with residual valvular damage. During the acute disease aspirin (80–100 mg/kg/day divided in 3–4 doses) or NSAIDs, particularly naproxen (20 mg/kg/day divided in 2 doses, maximum 500 mg twice daily) is given until normalization of all acute phase reactants. Corticosteroid use is restricted to significant cardiac involvement, especially myocarditis, and is given for 2–3 weeks and then changed to aspirin/NSAIDs. Sports and strenuous physical activity are restricted until normalization of acute phase reactants and dependent on the

TABLE 11.2 Prophylactic antibiotic treatment to prevent streptococcal infection

Preferred	
Penicillin G benzathine	1.2 Million Units IM q 3–4 weeks[a] 600,000 Units IM q 3–4 weeks if ≤27 kg
Alternative	
Penicillin V	250 mg PO twice daily
If allergic to penicillin	
Erythromycin	250 mg PO twice daily
Sulfadiazine	500 mg PO once daily if ≤27 kg 1 g PO once daily if >27 kg

[a]Injection required every 3 weeks if there is cardiac involvement in an endemic region

cardiac function. The entire family and close contacts should undergo a throat culture.

11.2.8   Outcome

The major morbidity and mortality from ARF arises from valvular heart damage. The valvular lesions resolves in 80 % of patients who receive long-term antibiotic prophylaxis [8]. Recurrent ARF is characterized with an increased incidence of severe carditis. Jaccoud arthropathy may be a rare long-term sequela.

11.3   Post-Streptococcal Reactive Arthritis (PSRA)

Post-streptococcal arthritis is a reactive arthritis that differs from the arthritis of ARF. It is non-migratory, lasts longer, does not respond as well to aspirin or NSAIDs, and typically involves both small and large joints [9–11]. Affected children do not have carditis or other major manifestations.

11.3.1   Epidemiology

There are no good epidemiologic studies of PSRA, but in North America it is more common than ARF. There are two peaks of incidence: late in childhood and early adolescence, and adults between 20 and 40 years of age, without a sex or ethnic predilection. It follows group A, C, and G streptococcal pharyngitis. It may be more common in children with HLA DRB1*01.

11.3.2   Clinical Manifestations

Most children with PSRA have additive and persistent poly-arthritis, frequently involving small joints of the fingers, although oligoarthritis and monoarthritis may occur. Axial disease may occur, more typically in those who are HLA-B27 positive. There is a shorter incubation period than ARF following the streptococcal infection (7–10 vs. 10–28 days, respectively).

11.3.3   Establishing the Diagnosis

The diagnosis requires evidence of prior streptococcal disease, the lack of major criteria for ARF, and non-migratory, non-fleeting arthritis. An mathematical model based on the acute phase reactants, response to therapy and recurrence of joint symptoms correctly classified >80 % of patients with ARF or PSRA [11].

11.3.4   Laboratory Features

Attempts to establish prior streptococcal disease as for ARF above should be made. Usually acute phase reactants are lower than in ARF. Additionally, we advocate searching for major and minor manifestations of ARF, especially obtaining an electrocardiogram and echocardiogram.

11.3.5   Treatment

Children with PSRA should be treated initially for streptococcus. Prophylaxis is controversial, since <5 % of children will have silent carditis and, over time may develop mitral regurgitation. Current recommendations are to give prophylactic antibiotics for 1 year and then, if an echocardiogram is normal, stop and watch carefully [7].

The arthritis is more persistent than that of ARF and not as responsive to NSAIDs, although NSAIDs do provide symptomatic relief. Intra-articular corticosteroids in those with a few joints involved will quickly resolve the arthritis in most. Some children will require a disease modifying agent, as in JIA (see Chap. 3). Physical therapy is beneficial in children with joint and muscle tightness.

11.3.6   Outcome

The arthritis of PSRA is longer lasting than ARF, but in most cases will resolve in 2–8 months. Recurrences of arthritis are more frequent than in ARF. Rarely children can have protracted arthritis.

References

1. Guidelines for the diagnosis of rheumatic fever. Jones Criteria, 1992 update. Special Writing Group of the Committee on Rheumatic Fever, Endocarditis, and Kawasaki Disease of the Council on Cardiovascular Disease in the Young of the American Heart Association. [Erratum in JAMA 1993;269:476]. JAMA. 1992;268:2069–73.
2. Amigo MC, Martinez-Lavin M, Reyes PA. Acute rheumatic fever. Rheum Dis Clin N Am. 1993;19:333–50.
3. Tani LY, Veasey LG, Minigill LL, et al. Rheumatic fever in children younger than 5 years: is the presentation different? Pediatrics. 2003;112:1065–8.

4. Bisno AL, Brito MO, Collins CM. Molecular basis of group A streptococcal virulence. Lancet Infect Dis. 2003;3:191–200.
5. Harel L, Zehana A, Kodman Y, et al. Presence of the D8/17 B-cell marker in children with rheumatic fever in Israel. Clin Genet. 2002;61:293–8.
6. Bonthius DJ, Karacay B. Sydenham's chorea: not gone and not forgotten. Semin Pediatr Neurol. 2003;10:11–9.
7. Gerber MA, Baltimore RS, Eaton CB, et al. Prevention of rheumatic fever and diagnosis and treatment of acute Streptococcal pharyngitis: a scientific statement from the American Heart Association Rheumatic Fever, Endocarditis, and Kawasaki Disease Committee of the Council on Cardiovascular Disease in the Young, the Interdisciplinary Council on Functional Genomics and Translational Biology, and the Interdisciplinary Council on Quality of Care and Outcomes Research: endorsed by the American Academy of Pediatrics. Circulation. 2009;119:1541–51.
8. Feldman T. Rheumatic heart disease. Curr Opin Cardiol. 1996;11:126–30.
9. Shulman ST, Ayoub EM. Poststreptococcal reactive arthritis. Curr Opin Rheumatol. 2002;14:562–5.
10. Uziel Y, Perl L, Barash J, Hashkes PJ. Post-streptococcal reactive arthritis in children: a distinct entity from acute rheumatic fever. Pediatr Rheumatol Online J. 2011;9:32.
11. Barash J, Mashiach E, Navon-Elkan P, et al. Differentiation of post streptococcal reactive arthritis from acute rheumatic fever. J Pediatr. 2008;153:696–9.

Chapter 12
Noninflammatory Mechanical Pain Syndromes

12.1 Introduction

Musculoskeletal pain is the presenting complaint in about 20 % of physician visits. Most complaints are short-lived and resolve uneventfully. We will discuss four major categories in this section, because they may mimic rheumatic conditions, or may come to the rheumatologist due to the perplexing nature of the condition for diagnosis and treatment, or are associated with significant morbidity. These include mechanical conditions (mostly orthopedic), the amplified musculoskeletal pain syndromes (see Chap. 13), and hereditary syndromes and tumors involving the musculoskeletal system (see Chaps. 14 and 15).

12.2 Benign Hypermobility Syndrome (BHMS)

Up to 20 % of girls are hypermobile, as are 10 % of boys. Adult patients with hypermobility, as defined by Beighton, usually have 5–6 out of 9 possible abnormalities on examination and this has been validated for Dutch children (Table 12.1; Figs. 12.1, 12.2, 12.3, 12.4, 12.5, 12.6, and 12.7) [1]. Children with pain due to benign hypermobility syndrome usually complain of pain in the evening, or at night

R.M. Laxer et al., *Pediatric Rheumatology in Clinical Practice*, 227
DOI 10.1007/978-3-319-13099-6_12,
© Springer-Verlag London 2016

TABLE 12.1 Beighton scale for hypermobility[a] [1]

	Score
Able to easily touch thumb to forearm, right and left	2
Hyperextend fifth MCP so finger parallels forearm, right and left	2
Greater than 10° hyperextension of elbows, right and left	2
Greater than 10° hyperextension of knees, right and left	2
Able to touch palms to floor with knees straight	1

[a]A score of five-six (preferably six) or more define hypermobility

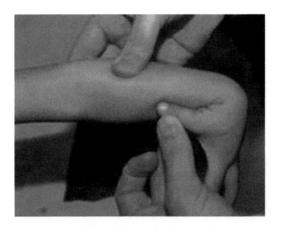

FIGURE 12.1 Demonstration of hypermobile thumb

after going to bed [2]. The pain can awaken the child and can be severe enough to cause crying and screaming. It is usually located in the legs, frequently behind the knee and is helped by massage, mild analgesics, and warmth. It is relatively short lived and most notable, the child is without stiffness or complaint in the morning and there is no gelling (stiffness after rest, such as a nap or long car ride). This is similar to the presentation of so called "growing pains" of childhood. The symptomatic child with BHMS often has

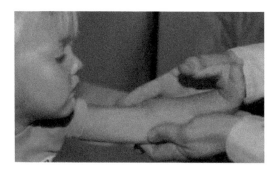

FIGURE 12.2 Demonstration of hypermobile MCPs

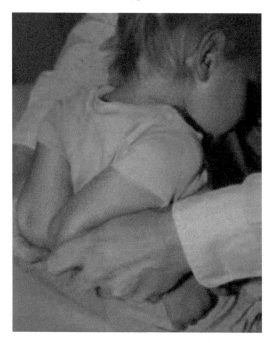

FIGURE 12.3 Demonstration of hypermobile shoulders

poor neuromuscular control. Asymmetric hypermobility in the weight bearing joints (e.g., hypermobile knees and not hips or ankles) can also lead to similar symptoms.

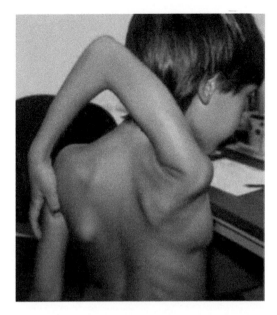

FIGURE 12.4 Demonstration of extremely hypermobile shoulders

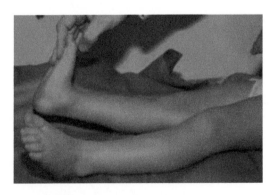

FIGURE 12.5 Demonstration of hypermobile knees

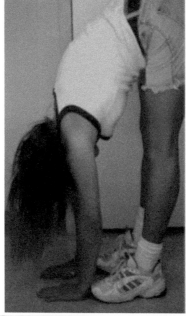

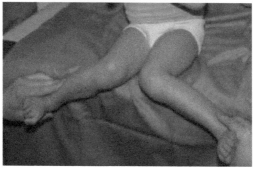

FIGURE 12.6 Demonstration of hypermobile hips

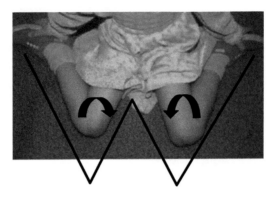

FIGURE 12.7 Demonstration of hypermobile hips and knees sitting in W position

The examination is notable only for hypermobility, and joint swelling is not usually present, although some patients with hypermobility can develop episodic noninflammatory joint swelling. The typical age for BHMS is 3–8 years, it is rare in adolescents and most children thought to have growing pain in the older age range usually have enthesitis (see Chap. 3). Features of Marfan syndrome and Ehlers–Danlos syndrome should be sought in any patient with hypermobility, since further consultation would be indicated. Some classify typical BHMS as described above, as Ehlers–Danlos type III. However, the more serious forms of Ehlers–Danlos syndrome are characterised by extreme hypermobility, loose skin (check over the forehead and sternum as well as the elbows and knees) (Fig. 12.8) and thin, cigarette paper scars [3]. Marfan syndrome is notable for arachnodactyly, high arched palate, long arms (the arm span times 1.03 is greater than the height), small elbow flexion contractures, disproportional long lower body segment, pectus carinatum or excavatum, and sparse subcutaneous body fat [4]. Children with other than type III Ehlers-Danlos should have a genetic consultation and many require surveillance for aortic dilation and aneurysms, and cardiac or ophthalmologic complications.

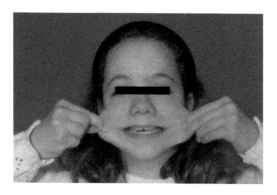

FIGURE 12.8 Exceptionally elastic skin of a girl with Ehlers–Danlos syndrome

The treatment of hypermobility is reassurance and, if pain is frequent, an evening dose of either acetaminophen, ibuprofen or longer lasting naproxen (for those children who awaken at night) can dramatically improve the evening life of the family. Parents should be warned to acknowledge the pain and give some measure of comfort (massage, reassurance to the child), but not unnecessary secondary gain (stories, sleeping with the parents, facilitating bedtime avoidance). Progressive exercises to improve balance and muscle strength/ control of the hypermobile joints are beneficial, as are orthotics in children with severe pes planus.

Some children with typical hypermobility pain are not hypermobile. These children have often been labelled as having "growing pains", although this term is a misnomer as it has nothing to do with the rate of growth. The cause of these pains are not clear but they may represent a pain amplification syndrome (see Chap. 13) or overuse pains. It is worth checking whether the symptomatic joint is next to a hypermobile joint, as this could often put undue stress on the nonhypermobile joint. The treatment is the same as for hypermobility, but it is important to repeat the musculoskeletal examination in 3–5 months to make sure subclinical illness has not evolved into arthritis or enthesitis.

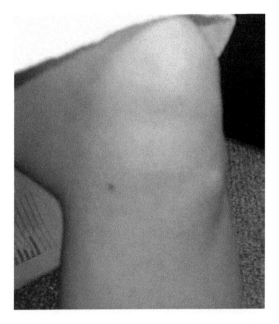

FIGURE 12.9 In Osgood–Schlatter disease, the tendon is thickened, often associated with a bursa and a very tender and enlarged tibial tubercle

12.3   Osgood–Schlatter Syndrome

Osgood–Schlatter syndrome is due to microavulsion fractures of the tibial tubercle, which is a secondary ossification center of the proximal tibia. The infrapatellar tendon pulls on the relative weak tibial tubercle enthesis leading to microavulsion. The bone remodels as the tendon continues to pull so a noticeable bump forms at the tibial tubercle (Fig. 12.9). It occurs in the rapidly growing adolescent, usually 8–13 years old. Boys outnumber girls 3:1. Patients with Osgood-Schlatter syndrome are very tender over the tibial tubercle and frequently are unable to kneel. It is bilateral in 30 % (Fig. 12.9). Treatment is rest and symptomatic care. The diagnosis is made clinically, but if severe and unremitting, a radiograph can ascertain if a pseudoarthrosis has formed, which will need surgical attention [5].

12.4 Sinding–Larsen–Johansson Syndrome

An analogous situation to Osgood–Schlatter syndrome can occur at the inferior pole of the patella, called Sinding–Larsen–Johansson syndrome. It, too, is more frequent in early adolescent boys, especially athletes. It is exacerbated by running, stairs and kneeling, and there is usually swelling. The treatment is rest and symptomatic care. In severe cases, a cast or splint can help enforce rest and hasten healing.

12.5 Sever Syndrome

Sever syndrome is an apophysitis of the calcaneus, usually in children aged 8–13 years. It is more common in boys by a 2:1 margin and causes activity related heel pain. It is characterized by point tenderness at the corner of the calcaneus. Heel cups help most of the time and, if needed, acetaminophen or ibuprofen may be administered.

12.6 Osteonecrosis

Children are susceptible to idiopathic osteonecrosis in a variety of bones. These may be due to trauma to the growing bone or in some cases to avascular necrosis. Eponyms are frequently used, depending on the location. The more common areas of osteonecrosis involve the hip (Legg–Calvé–Perthes, discussed below), lunate (Kienböck), second metatarsal head (Freiberg), proximal tibia (Blount), tarsal navicular (Köhler), and vertebral epiphysis (Scheuermann). Treatment is usually supportive and may require temporary splinting and avoiding activities that lead to trauma to the area involved (such as karate with Kienböck).

12.7   Costochondritis

One of the most common causes of chest pain in older adolescents is costochondritis, inflammation of the cartilaginous junction of the rib and sternum. It is more common in girls. It is termed Tietze syndrome if swelling is present. It is usually post viral and can last for months. It is aggravated with trauma and even from lying prone on a hard surface, such as reading while on the floor.

12.8   Epicondylitis

Point tenderness of the medial epicondyle (golfer's or little league elbow) or lateral epicondyle (tennis elbow) is an overuse injury seen in adolescent athletes. It causes local pain and is characterised by point tenderness that increases with resisted motion. Conservative measures, such as ice, counterforce bracing, and rest usually suffice, although some patients need NSAIDs or local corticosteroid injection.

12.9   Hip Pain

Isolated hip pain is of special urgency due to the inability to feel joint swelling, the susceptibility of the hip to various conditions and infection, and the importance of hip in function [6]. Differential diagnoses include the following:

12.9.1   Septic Hip/Osteomyelitis

Septic arthritis of the hip is not uncommon and requires intravenous antibiotics and drainage. It is most common below the age of 5; boys outnumber girls 2:1. *Staphylococcus aureus* is the most common organism. It causes severe acute pain and usually causes immobility of the hip and prevents

weight bearing. It is accompanied by fever, malaise, and elevated acute phase reactants. It is usually not confused with
the rheumatic or mechanical conditions, although an occasional child with oligoarthritis of the hip, toxic/transient synovitis, reactive arthritis also enthesitis-related arthritis, chronic
recurrent multifocal osteomyelitis or acute rheumatic fever
will need to be investigated for potential septic hip.

12.9.2   *Toxic Synovitis (Transient Synovitis, Observation Hip)*

Toxic synovitis affecting the hip is more common in boys
aged 3–10 years, and frequently follows an upper respiratory
tract infection. It is neither as painful, nor as limiting of
mobility, as is a septic hip, and the acute phase reactants are
normal or only mildly elevated. If infection is suspected, joint
aspiration is indicated. Normally it can be treated with
NSAIDs and rest over time. Most symptoms resolve within a
week. Frequent recurrence should alert the physician to
evolving enthesitis-related arthritis.

12.10   Legg–Calvé–Perthes

Legg–Calvé–Perthes is an avascular necrosis of the femoral head usually seen in children aged 4–10 years. It is
more frequent in boys, 4:1, and is bilateral in 20 %. The
presenting complaint is frequently a painless limp. It is
diagnosed early by MRI and later by plain radiography,
and there are five radiologic stages: (1) cessation of capital femoral epiphyseal growth, (2) subchondral fracture,
(3) resorption (fragmentation), (4) reossification, and (5)
healed or residual stage (Fig. 12.10). It is a self-limited
condition and the goal of treatment is to contain the
femoral head within the acetabulum so that the latter acts
as a mold, preventing further long-term damage.
Orthopedic expertise should be obtained early. Prognosis

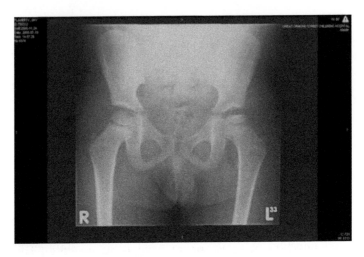

FIGURE 12.10 Legg–Calvé–Perthes of the left hip

is based primarily on the age of onset, with younger children doing much better, and secondarily the degree of femoral head collapse [7].

12.11   Slipped Capital Femoral Epiphysis

Slipped capital femoral epiphysis (SCFE) is a fracture through the femoral head epiphysis. SCFE occurs most frequently in obese adolescents, but can also afflict those who have delayed skeletal maturation, or who are tall and thin with a recent growth spurt. It may have an underlying endocrinologic cause, especially hypothyroidism. It can have an acute or chronic onset, so it may not present as an acutely painful hip. A new limp with limited internal rotation of the hip should prompt radiographs, anteriorposterior and frog leg lateral projections. Widening of the physis without slippage is the earliest sign of SCFE, but as the slip progresses, the head remains in the acetabulum and the femoral neck rotates downward and anteriorly. Urgent orthopedic consultation is indicated.

12.12   Idiopathic Chondrolysis of the Hip

Idiopathic chondrolysis is characterised by progressive loss of cartilage in adolescents, affects more girls than boys and has a slight predilection in Africans and African Americans. The diagnosis is made radiographically, with the exclusion of other conditions, usually requiring biopsy. Treatment is symptomatic and ultimately surgical.

12.13   Laboratory Tests

In children presenting with most of the above conditions, no laboratory tests are indicated. If there is concern about an early infection then acute phase reactants (CBC, ESR, CRP) should be checked. Rheumatologic disease laboratory studies are usually not indicated. Fifteen percent of normal children will have a nonspecific positive ANA test that will lead to unnecessary referral, expense, and worry [8].

Imaging studies are universally required for hip symptoms since SCFE needs immediate attention and Legg–Calvé–Perthes needs orthopedic treatment, not anti-inflammatory treatment. Other radiographs are indicated if osteonecrosis or trauma is suspected. Radiographs do not help with the early identification of arthritis although many rheumatologists like to establish a baseline to compare to subsequent studies to determine the rate of joint damage. Ultrasound, scintigraphy and MRI have their place and are discussed when indicated throughout this text.

References

1. Beighton P, Solomon L, Soskolne CL. Articular mobility in an African population. Ann Rheum Dis. 1973;32:413–8.
2. Viswanathan V, Khubchandani RP. Joint hypermobility and growing pains in school children. Clin Exp Rheumatol. 2008;26:962–6.
3. Sobey G. Ehlers-Danlos syndrome: how to diagnose and when to perform genetic tests. Arch Dis Child. 2015;100:57–61.

4. Faivre L, Collod-Beroud G, Ades L, et al. The new Ghent criteria for Marfan syndrome: what do they change? Clin Genet. 2012;81:433–42.
5. Gholve PA, Scher DM, Khakharia S, et al. Osgood Schlatter syndrome. Curr Opin Pediatr. 2007;19:44–50.
6. Cook PC. Transient synovitis, septic hip, and Legg-Calve-Perthes disease: an approach to the correct diagnosis. Pediatr Clin North Am. 2014;61:1109–18.
7. Chaudhry S, Phillips D, Feldman D. Legg-Calve-Perthes disease: an overview with recent literature. Bull Hosp Jt Dis. 2014;72:18–27.
8. Wananukul S, Voramethkul W, Kaewopas Y, Hanvivatvong O. Prevalence of positive antinuclear antibodies in healthy children. Asian Pac J Allergy Immunol. 2005;23:153–7.

Chapter 13
Amplified Musculoskeletal Pain

13.1 Introduction

An increasing number of children have various forms of amplified musculoskeletal pain. These children are often more disabled than children with arthritis and they and their families suffer intensely. In addition to their pain, frequently they are isolated from peers and are commonly told by medical professionals that they are faking it or that it does not hurt all that much. Treating these children is very challenging but quite rewarding.

13.2 Definition

Chronic musculoskeletal pain increased out of proportion to the known stimulus.

13.2.1 Nomenclature

There are multiple manifestations of amplified musculoskeletal pain, usually defined by the location or presence of autonomic dysfunction. Two broad categories of amplified musculoskeletal pain are localised pain and diffuse [1]. Of those with localised pain, the most easily recognised is

R.M. Laxer et al., *Pediatric Rheumatology in Clinical Practice*,   241
DOI 10.1007/978-3-319-13099-6_13,
© Springer-Verlag London 2016

complex regional pain syndrome type (CRPS), formerly known as reflex sympathetic dystrophy [2]. These children have overt autonomic dysfunction manifest by coolness or cyanosis of the limb and occasionally increased perspiration or edema. Many children have very localized pain amplification but do not have autonomic signs. Of the children with diffuse pain, the most well-known is fibromyalgia. The criteria for fibromyalgia have evolved over the years and the 2010 American College of Rheumatology criteria seems as reliable in adolescents as the earlier published criteria and do not require tender point examination [3–5]. Fibromyalgia requires 3 months of widespread pain and as well as a measure of the degree of symptom severity (Table 13.1). However, many children can be classified as having two pain syndromes (CRPS and fibromyalgia) or do not meet criteria for either due to lack of associated symptoms or the intermittent nature of the pain. Figure 13.1 shows the overlapping nature of the various pain syndromes.

13.3   Epidemiology

There are no specific studies of the incidence of amplified musculoskeletal pain in children. Studies of normal school-children have found 1.2–6 % fulfil criteria for fibromyalgia and 7.5 % report widespread musculoskeletal pain. Children with amplified musculoskeletal pain make up approximately 10 % of children in pediatric rheumatic disease clinics and it is the impression of many that the incidence is increasing [6, 7].

The average age of onset is preteen to early adolescence. It is rare below the age of 7 years so diagnosing amplified musculoskeletal pain in young children needs to be done with much circumspection. However, children as young as 2 and 3 years old have developed amplified pain.

Girls are overrepresented at a ratio of at least 5:1. This may be because girls have lower pain thresholds and report pain more frequently than boys. However, others have

TABLE 13.1 A modification of the 2010 American College of Rheumatology criteria for fibromyalgia

All 3 conditions must be satisfied:

1. Absence of a disorder to explain the pain

2. Symptoms present for 3 months

3. One of the below

  a. Widespread pain index ≥7 and symptom severity score ≥5

  b. Widespread pain index 3–6 and symptom severity score ≥9

Widespread pain index calculated by adding number of body regions in pain within the last week including: jaw, shoulder, upper arm, lower arm, buttocks, upper leg, lower leg (2 points if bilateral) and single points for neck, chest, abdomen, upper back and lower back [total possible score 19]

Symptom severity score be as high as 12 and is calculated by adding the sum of the self-reported severity scores for 3 core symptoms: fatigue, waking unrefreshed and thinking difficulty (0 = no problem, 1 = mild problem, 2 = moderate problem, 3 = severe problem [total possible score 9] and a symptom checklist score, 0 = no symptoms, 1 = 1–10 symptoms, 2 = 11–24 symptoms, 3 = 25+ symptoms [total possible score 3]

The symptoms may include: muscle pain, headaches, tiredness, muscle weakness, abdominal pain, nausea, nervousness, dizziness, thinking problems, irritable bowel symptoms (bloating, gas, intermittent diarrhea/constipation), chest pain, insomnia – getting or staying asleep, easy bruising, depression, ringing in ears, numbness, dry mouth, loss of appetite, heartburn, blurry vision, shortness of breath, frequent urination, dry eyes, itching, Raynaud – hands or feet with color changes, ongoing constipation, ongoing diarrhea, oral ulcers, hair loss, loss of taste or change of taste, hearing difficulties, wheezing, vomiting, bladder spasms, painful urination, hives/welts, seizures, sun sensitivity, light sensitivity other than sun sensitivity, noise sensitivity, sensitivity to strong smells, seeing spots, partial or total blindness, double vision, difficulty reading, lightheadedness or feeling woozy, balance problems, fainting or near fainting, heart racing/palpitations, uncontrollable shaking of muscles, twitching of muscles or tics, inability to move part of your body/paralysis, part of your body so stiff it cannot bend or move, reversal of day/night sleep wake cycle, severe menstrual cramps

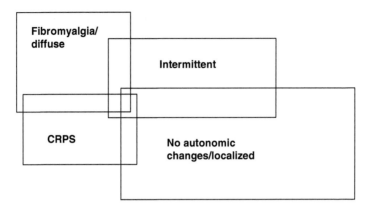

FIGURE 13.1 The overlapping nature of the various forms of amplified musculoskeletal pain in children. Not all children with diffuse pain satisfy the criteria for fibromyalgia. Additionally, there are children with intermittent localized or diffuse pains or overlapping features of the above, e.g., a cool blue foot and total body pain

reported that boys and girls with chronic pain do not differ in physician utilization.

Most children with amplified musculoskeletal pain are Caucasian, however, no race or economic level is spared.

13.4   Etiology

The etiology is unknown but it seems related to trauma, illness, or psychological distress. The trauma is usually mild but occasionally is more severe such as a fracture. It can follow acute and chronic illnesses that are associated with pain such as viral syndromes, sickle cell anemia, inflammatory bowel disease, arthritis, or other rheumatic illnesses. Most pediatric rheumatologists think that psychological distress plays a significant role in most, but not all cases [8–10]. Whether cause or effect, in most children the pain and dysfunction themselves inflicts psychological havoc on the child and family. Genetic factors have been implicated in fibromyalgia and

CRPS and a weak association has been made between fibromyalgia and hypermobility (see Chap. 12). It is likely that a combination of both intrinsic factors, such as individual pain threshold, female sex, and coping strategies and extrinsic factors, such as previous pain experiences, social stresses, modeling of chronic pain behaviors, and central and peripheral pain mechanisms work in concert to give rise to amplified musculoskeletal pain [8].

13.5 Clinical Manifestations

Although each child is different, there are unifying threads in the history and physical examination to establish the pattern for most. The archetypal patient is a mature and accomplished adolescent girl who suffers a minor injury or illness and then has increasing pain and dysfunction over several days to months. The pain may be localised, with or without signs of autonomic dysfunction, or diffuse. Sometimes it begins as localised pain and spreads. Allodynia is common and minimal trauma such as clothing, bumps while riding in the car, and even the wind hitting the skin causes pain. Some children, usually those with diffuse pain, will have multiple somatic complaints, which help define fibromyalgia (Table 13.1). The child will report very high levels of pain (10 out of 10) usually with an incongruent, cheerful affect and la belle indifference about the level of dysfunction. Like the pain, the amount of dysfunction is disproportionate and frequently leads to incapacitation. Multiple physician visits and therapeutic failures are common.

Autonomic signs seen in CRPS usually consist of coolness and cyanosis (Fig. 13.2). These signs may not be manifest at rest but become apparent after exercising the limb. Occasionally there is edema, increased perspiration or dystrophic skin (Fig. 13.3).

Allodynia is tested by either light touch or gentle pinching of a fold of skin. The area of allodynia usually varies in location on repeated testing.

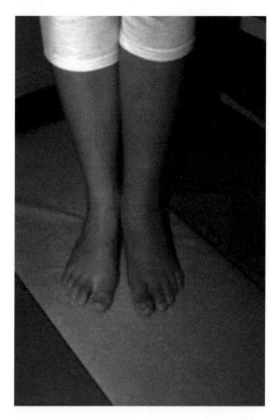

FIGURE 13.2 Cyanosis and slight swelling in an adolescent girl with CRPS of the left foot: it was extremely tender to light touch (allodynia)

Conversion symptoms are not infrequent; motor conversions are the most common and include the inability to move a limb or hand due to muscle contraction (not true dystonia), non-physiologic gait abnormalities, paralysis, or abnormal shaking, pseudoseizures or tremors. Sensory conversions such as dizziness and visual changes are also not uncommon.

Frequently is it evident that there exists an unusually close bond between the patient and parent, usually daughter and

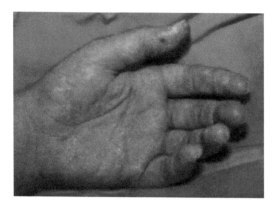

Figure 13.3 Dystrophic skin changes in an adolescent with CRPS

mother, in which the mother will be overly enmeshed with the child and the child's pain and disability. The mother can feel the pain and in trying to be compassionate and nurturing actually enables the child to be disabled and overly dependent. The pain controls not only the child but the entire family.

13.6   Laboratory Tests

All laboratory blood and urine tests are normal. Low vitamin D levels are associated with increased pain but correction of the deficit usually does not have a significant effect on the pain [11]. Radiographs may show osteoporosis and bone scintigraphy is usually normal but it can show decreased uptake, especially in CRPS (or spotty increased uptake characteristic of adult CRPS). Magnetic resonance images can show edema, but the anatomy is otherwise intact [12].

13.7   Diagnostic Pitfalls

It is essential to conduct a thorough physical examination as disorders such as spondyloarthropathy and spinal cord tumors can present with non-specific pain that can be confused as an amplified pain syndrome. The presence of enthesitis can be overlooked if not checked for specifically (Chap. 3). Arthritis has been mistaken for amplified musculoskeletal pain, but it is usually obvious on examination. Some children with arthritis will also have, amplified musculoskeletal pain syndrome so both disorders need to be addressed.

13.8   Disease Activity

Initially and during follow-up, there needs to be ongoing assessment of pain and dysfunction. Self-report, such as 0–10 on a verbal scale or marking a visual analogue scale, is adequate to measure pain. Functional measures usually consist of a questionnaire inquiring about a standard set of age-appropriate activities, but, in practice, asking about school attendance, walking endurance, chores and participation in recreational activities will suffice.

13.9   Treatment

It is paramount to establish a trusting relationship with the child and family. Foremost, caregivers need to acknowledge that the pain is real since these children have been given both verbal and nonverbal messages that the pain is all in their head or that they are malingering. It is useful to explain the pain in terms of sympathetically mediated pain amplification (Fig. 13.4); this reinforces the reality of the pain, gives an understandable reason for the pain, and is a mechanism in which to introduce the treatment strategy [13].

It is essential to be confident in the diagnosis and to stop doing medical investigations. Families are often convinced that some diagnosis has been overlooked and that a test (even if done previously and was normal) will establish a more tangible or familiar diagnosis.

All analgesic medications should be discontinued. Some children who are on medications for depression or anxiety will need to continue, but those treated with

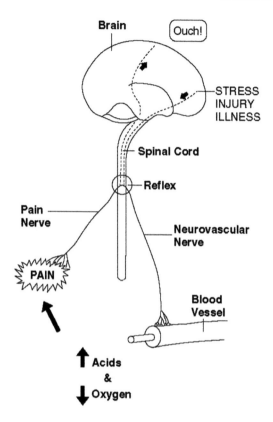

FIGURE 13.4 Working model to explain amplified musculoskeletal pain via sympathetically mediated tissue ischemia

antidepressants for pain should stop taking the drug. Some medications need to be tapered, specifically, opioids should be tapered about 10 % a day and gabapentin over 2–3 weeks, depending on the dose. Tramadol binds to μ opioid receptors so, if on a high dose, it should also be tapered.

There are no controlled studies of the vast number of reported treatments for the various forms of amplified musculoskeletal pain. Treatments have ranged from pain medications, antidepressants, gabapentin, transcutaneous nerve stimulation, nerve blocks and sympathectomy (for CRPS), epidural catheters for continuous infusion including pain pumps, lidocaine and opioid patches, acupuncture, cognitive-behavior therapy, psychotherapy, and exercise therapy.

Most agree that exercise therapy is helpful and it is associated with the best long-term outcomes in all forms of amplified musculoskeletal pain and we have found it the most helpful with the longest lasting results [14, 15]. The nature of the exercise therapy is different to that which most physical and occupational therapists are accustomed to. The primary goal is to restore function so the program is very intense and directed at doing normal and aerobic activities, such as jumping, stairs, walking speed and endurance, sports drills, and carrying loads. Pain is not directly treated and is ignored as much as possible during the exercising. The vast majority will resolve all pain once full function has been restored. Allodynia is treated with desensitization with towel and lotion rubs. Many children will require up to 5 hours of exercise therapy daily, on average, for 2–3 weeks. Additionally, most children will show improvement in their mood, sleep, energy level, and other somatic complaints.

In addition to exercise, the psychodynamics of the child and family should be evaluated, since most families and children, but not all, will have significant psychological problems that can be helped with individual, family, or marital therapy [10, 14, 16]. Consultation with a mental health professional is often extremely helpful.

Sleep deserves special mention, but addressing sleep problems does not resolve the somatic symptoms. Many children with amplified musculoskeletal pain have a sleep complaint (not a true sleep disorder) and good sleep hygiene is helpful. This includes going to bed only when one is sleepy, not engaging in other activities in bed such as reading or watching television, using computers or smartphones, eliminating caffeine, relaxation techniques, elimination of napping and having a routine for sleeping and waking. After an intense exercise program, most children with fibromyalgia slept well [17].

Traditional (nonallopathic) treatments are frequently sought, but there are no data regarding benefit in children. Tai chi and pilates may help some adults with fibromyalgia and qigong has been shown in children to not exacerbate the pain [18]. These traditional therapies include herbal therapy, massage, magnet therapy, homeopathy, reflexology, and aromatherapy to name a few, but only rarely is any sustained benefit reported. We cannot recommend any and, like allopathic medications, we discontinue them once the diagnosis is clear.

13.10   Outcome

The outcome may vary on the form of amplified musculoskeletal pain; however, long-term studies in children are few. Most children (92 % in one series of 103 children) with CRPS treated with an intense exercise program resolved all signs and symptoms and 88 % were well after 5 years [15]. These results have been replicated by others [19, 20]. Children with diffuse pain or fibromyalgia may have more long-term pain, depending on the treatment and study [14, 16]. However, of 64 children with fibromyalgia treated with intense exercise therapy and counseling, at 1 year half had pain scores measured as ≤1/10 [14].

Children with amplified musculoskeletal pain may go on to develop other sites of chronic pain such as headaches and abdominal pain [21]. Additionally, other outcomes not associated with the pain itself may take on many forms of unresolved psychological issues and include conversion reactions, eating disorders, school avoidance, suicide attempts, and acting out behaviors.

13.11   Summary

Children with amplified musculoskeletal pain suffer significant pain and disability and need compassionate care that should include accurate diagnosis, as well as a consistent evaluative and therapeutic approach. The psychological aspects of these conditions should be formally assessed. Intense exercise therapy, along with desensitisation, is of great benefit to most. Normal function should be restored at a minimum. School attendance should be mandatory and social activities and sports encouraged. If pain continues, then either pain coping skills using cognitive behavioral therapy, or more formal psychotherapy should be pursued. Pharmacological agents should be limited to specific indications, not pain control. Treating children with amplified musculoskeletal pain and their families can be challenging, but the benefit gained by all is quite rewarding.

Key Points

Have a high index of suspicion for the presence of amplified musculoskeletal pain especially in:

- Adolescent girls
- Mature beyond years
- Accomplished
- Perfectionistic
- Pleaser
- Prolonged school absence due to pain
- Marked dysfunction
- Pain is continuing to get worse
- Normal examination except pain
- No enthesitis or arthritis
- Normal neurological exam
- Normal laboratory studies
- Failure of all prior therapies

  Localised pain on examination

- Allodynia (variable border)
- Autonomic signs
- Incongruent affect
- La belle indifference

  Widespread pain on examination

- Allodynia (variable border)
- Total body allodynia (although frequently spares palms, soles, breasts and genitals)

- Nonorganic back signs
- Incongruent affect

Once an amplified musculoskeletal pain is recognized acknowledge the pain and explain that it is amplified, not indicative of underlying damage or disease

- Stop further medical investigations
- Stop medications for pain
- Restore function

Aerobic exercise, up to 5 h daily of intense therapy focused on functional activities that may take 2–3 weeks. If allodynia is present, desensitize with tactile stimulation.

- Resume full school attendance
- Resume social and recreational activities
- Have the psychological dynamics evaluated and appropriately treated
- Anticipate total resolution of symptoms, not just coping or control

References

1. Malleson PN, al-Matar M, Petty RE. Idiopathic musculoskeletal pain syndromes in children. J Rheumatol. 1992;19:1786–9.
2. Merskey H, Bogduk N. Classification of chronic pain: descriptions of chronic pain syndromes and definitions of pain terms. 2nd ed. Seattle: IASP press; 1994.
3. Yunus MB, Masi AT. Juvenile primary fibromyalgia syndrome. A clinical study of thirty-three patients and matched normal controls. Arthritis Rheum. 1985;28:138–45.
4. Wolfe F, Clauw DJ, Fitzcharles MA, et al. The American College of Rheumatology preliminary diagnostic criteria for fibromyalgia and measurement of symptom severity. Arthritis Care Res (Hoboken). 2010;62:600–10.
5. Ting TV, Barnett K, Lynch-Jordan A, Whitacre C, Henrickson M, Kashikar-Zuck S. American College of Rheumatology Adult Fibromyalgia Criteria for use in an adolescent female population with juvenile fibromyalgia. J Pediatr. 2016;169:181–7.

6. Bowyer S, Roettcher P. Pediatric rheumatology clinic populations in the United States: results of a 3 year survey. Pediatric Rheumatology Database Research Group. J Rheumatol. 1996;23:1968–74.

7. Malleson PN, Fung MY, Rosenberg AM. The incidence of pediatric rheumatic diseases: results from the Canadian Pediatric Rheumatology Association Disease Registry. J Rheumatol. 1996;23:1981–7.

8. Bernstein BH, Singsen BH, Kent JT, et al. Reflex neurovascular dystrophy in childhood. J Pediatr. 1978;93:211–5.

9. Kashikar-Zuck S, Parkins IS, Graham TB, et al. Anxiety, mood, and behavioral disorders among pediatric patients with juvenile fibromyalgia syndrome. Clin J Pain. 2008;24:620–6.

10. Sherry DD, Weisman R. Psychologic aspects of childhood reflex neurovascular dystrophy. Pediatrics. 1988;81:572–8.

11. Straube S, Derry S, Straube C, Moore RA. Vitamin D for the treatment of chronic painful conditions in adults. Cochrane Database Syst Rev. 2015;5, CD007771.

12. Schurmann M, Zaspel J, Lohr P, et al. Imaging in early posttraumatic complex regional pain syndrome: a comparison of diagnostic methods. Clin J Pain. 2007;23:449–57.

13. Sherry DD. An overview of amplified musculoskeletal pain syndromes. J Rheum Suppl. 2000;58:44–8.

14. Sherry DD, Brake L, Tress JL, et al. The treatment of juvenile fibromyalgia with an intensive physical and psychosocial program. J Pediatr. 2015;167:731–7.

15. Sherry DD, Wallace CA, Kelley C, et al. Short- and long-term outcomes of children with complex regional pain syndrome type I treated with exercise therapy. Clin J Pain. 1999;15:218–23.

16. Kashikar-Zuck S, Ting TV, Arnold LM, et al. Cognitive behavioral therapy for the treatment of juvenile fibromyalgia: a multisite, single-blind, randomized, controlled clinical trial. Arthritis Rheum. 2012;64:297–305.

17. Olsen MN, Sherry DD, Boyne K, et al. Relationship between sleep and pain in adolescents with juvenile primary fibromyalgia syndrome. Sleep. 2013;36:509–16.

18. Stephens S, Feldman BM, Bradley N, et al. Feasibility and effectiveness of an aerobic exercise program in children with fibromyalgia: results of a randomized controlled pilot trial. Arthritis Rheum. 2008;59:1399–406.

19. Brooke V, Janselewitz S. Outcomes of children with complex regional pain syndrome after intensive inpatient rehabilitation. Phys Med Rehabil. 2012;4:349–54.
20. Logan DE, Carpino EA, Chiang G, et al. A day-hospital approach to treatment of pediatric complex regional pain syndrome: initial functional outcomes. Clin J Pain. 2012;28: 766–74.
21. Sherry DD. Amplified musculoskeletal pain: treatment approach and outcomes. J Pediatr Gastroenterol Nutr. 2008;47:693–4.

Chapter 14
Hereditary Conditions of Bone and Cartilage

14.1   Introduction

Generalized genetic disorders of bone and cartilage growth and development are called skeletal dysplasias or osteochondrodysplasias. The International Nosology and Classification of Constitutional Disorders of Bone (ninth edition, 2015) identified 436 different skeletal dysplasias that were classified based on molecular, biochemical and radiographic criteria [1]. Also included in the classification are the dysostoses (because there is often clinical overlap with the skeletal dysplasias) and disorders of bone mineralization. The classification identifies three major groups of dysostoses, those with predominant facial and cranial disorders, those with predominant axial involvement, and those with predominant involvement of the extremities. Many are associated with extra-osseous features that characterize the phenotype and help with accurate diagnosis.

14.2   Epidemiology

The overall group has a prevalence of between 250 and 350 per million in the population.

R.M. Laxer et al., *Pediatric Rheumatology in Clinical Practice*,   257
DOI 10.1007/978-3-319-13099-6_14,
© Springer-Verlag London 2016

14.3   Clinical Features

Patients are often considered to have juvenile idiopathic arthritis (JIA) based on musculoskeletal restrictions and deformities. Features that help differentiate JIA from the hereditary disorders of cartilage and bone are listed in Table 14.1 [2].

There is often a family history of musculoskeletal problems. Clinical signs include short stature, malformation/shortening of limbs, or dysmorphic features. Often the presentation is one of restriction of movements rather than pain. Pain and stiffness can affect joints as well as the spine. There is no evidence of inflammation. A skeletal survey shows the characteristic abnormalities in the epiphyses and in some, the metaphyses (Figs. 14.1, 14.2, and 14.3). In the dysostosis group, additional clues include the texture of the skin, especially the palms, tendon thickening and shortening (Fig. 14.4), a family history of premature osteoarthritis, perhaps requiring joint replacement, and consanguinity

Table 14.1 Features suggesting a diagnosis of a heritable disorder of cartilage or bone versus JIA

Bone deformities and restricted motion outweigh pain
Absence of laboratory signs of systemic inflammation
Family history often positive for similar disorder
Early onset of familial osteoarthritis with need for arthroplasty
Presence of hearing loss
Presence of vitreal and/or retinal disease
Presence of dysmorphic features
Generalized hypermobility
Congenital camptodactyly

Adapted from Chalom et al. [2]

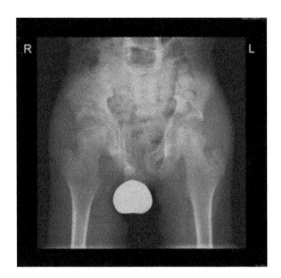

FIGURE 14.1 Pelvic radiograph of a child with Stickler syndrome, showing hypoplasia of iliac wings, thickened femoral neck, metaphyseal irregularities, flattening of femoral epiphysis, acetabular protrusio, and narrowed sciatic notch

within the family (for autosomal recessive disorders). It is important to search for clinical manifestations in tissues and organs that have the same proteins as the bones and joints as they may help establish a diagnosis (e.g., type II collagen abnormalities also involve the eye and ear; type XI collagen abnormalities involve the ear but not the eye). Additional examples of patients with mutations of structural proteins are shown in Figs. 14.5, 14.6, and 14.7.

14.4   Diagnosis

A skeletal survey should be obtained on presentation and before the closure of the epiphyses. A diagnosis may be made following identification of the major areas of bone

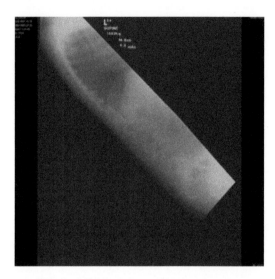

FIGURE 14.2 Spine radiograph of a child with multiple epiphyseal dysplasia, showing abnormal flattened vertebrae: He has a mutation in the matrillin-3 gene

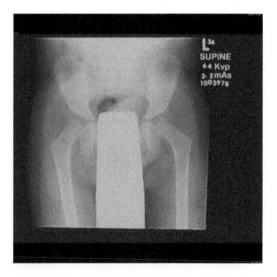

FIGURE 14.3 Pelvic radiograph of a child with multiple epiphyseal dysplasia with mutation in the matrillin-3 gene

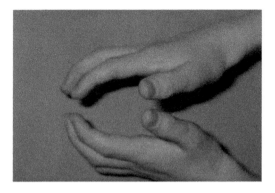

FIGURE 14.4 Hands of a child with mucolipidosis type III. Note the thickened tendons and inability to straighten the fingers

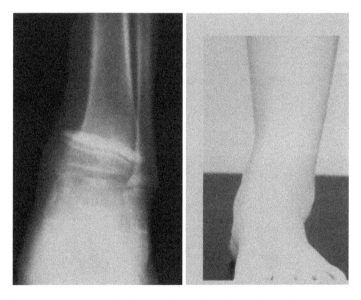

FIGURE 14.5 Clinical photograph and radiograph of a 10-year-old girl who presented with bilateral foot pain and malalignment: the AP view of the left ankle shows subphyseal metaphyseal sclerosis and ankle tilt consistent with metaphyseal fractures typical of idiopathic juvenile osteoporosis

abnormality, dislocations, overgrowth, pseudoarthroses, short ribs, and club feet. The final diagnosis will include a combination of findings and the name often incorporates the major areas affected—for example, 'craniodiaphyseal dysplasia', 'spondyloepiphyseal dysplasia', or 'acromesomelic dysplasia'. Recent advances in molecular genetics allow for genetic diagnoses to be made in many of these disorders. There are several databases that can assist with diagnosis (e.g. Online Mendelian Inheritance in Man, OMIM) [3].

14.5   Treatment

In the case of dysplasias, maintenance of function with physiotherapy and regular appropriate exercises are all that is necessary. Occasionally pain relief medication will be necessary.

In the case of dysostosis multiplex, supportive measures have been the only treatment option for the past decades. Specific enzyme/gene replacement therapies early in the presentation are promising for some of these disorders.

In the idiopathic osteolyses, bisphosphonates have been occasionally helpful in reducing pain associated with the osteolysis, but the renal impairment is not responsive.

14.6   Prognosis

A molecular genetic diagnosis is very helpful in predicting the course of the condition. The dysplasias vary in severity and therefore in the functional outcome, but there is usually no increase in mortality. The dysostosis multiplex group differs from the storage diseases in that patients with storage diseases are more prone to avascular necrosis in weight bearing joints and metabolic disease. Of the osteolysis syndromes, carpaltarsal osteolysis is often associated with renal impairment, as well as progressive functional impairment due to loss of wrist and ankle bones and shortening of phalanges.

14.7   Unique Disorders

Several diseases deserve special mention because early recognition can prevent unnecessary investigation or earlier intervention that can prevent longer-term complications. Joint hypermobility may occur on its own or as part of a clinical syndrome (See Chap. 12). The most common associations are with Marfan syndrome and Ehlers-Danlos syndrome.

14.7.1   Marfan Syndrome

Patients with Marfan syndrome have tall stature, upward dislocation of the lens, pectus excavatum (or sometimes carinatum), high-arched palate, arachnodactyly and are at risk for aortic root dissection; therefore screening by ophthalmology and cardiology is important. Mutations in the fibrillin 1 gene lead to Marfan syndrome which can be autosomal dominant or sporadic.

14.7.2   Ehlers-Danlos Syndromes

There are several types of Ehlers-Danlos syndromes with mutations in various collagen genes as well as other structural genes. They are classified based on the different clinical features which can include varying degrees of hyperlaxity of the skin and joint hypermobility (± joint dislocation), poor wound healing and easy bruising. Ehlers Danlos type IV is particularly severe as it is associated with vascular ruptures and ruptures of the hollow organs such as the stomach, intestine and uterus. Genetic analysis can help confirm the diagnosis.

14.7.3   Osteogenesis Imperfecta

Osteogenesis imperfecta may also be associated with hypermobile joints but its most important feature is the development of spontaneous fractures with minor or minimal trauma. There are several forms associated with mutations in *COL1A1*, *COL1A2*, *CRTAP*, and *P3H1*. The most severe form can present with intra-uterine fractures, but more commonly fractures occur when children begin to walk or may not occur until later childhood or adolescence. Back pain secondary to vertebral compression fractures may be the first sign of the disease.

14.7.4   Camptodactyly-Arthropathy-Coxa Vara-Pericarditis (CACP) Syndrome

CACP syndrome results from mutations in the proteoglycan-4 gene on chromosome 1q31 gene which codes for the protein lubricin. It is autosomal recessive in inheritance and there may be a history of parental consanguinity. Abnormalities in lubricin lead to loss of proper lubrication in tendon sheaths, synovial and serosal fluids. The clinical presentation is often confused with JIA as patients present with large joint effusions, especially around the knees, ankles and wrists. As opposed to JIA, there is often a history of "trigger fingers" present at birth or very early in life, and the swelling is non-inflammatory (Fig. 14.6). The joints are not warm or painful and there is no history of morning stiffness. With time, large intra-osseous cysts develop, especially in the acetabulae and coxa vara is seen radiologically (Fig. 14.7). Unfortunately there is no specific treatment that is beneficial other than physical therapy and trying to be as active as possible. Hip replacements are often indicated in early adulthood.

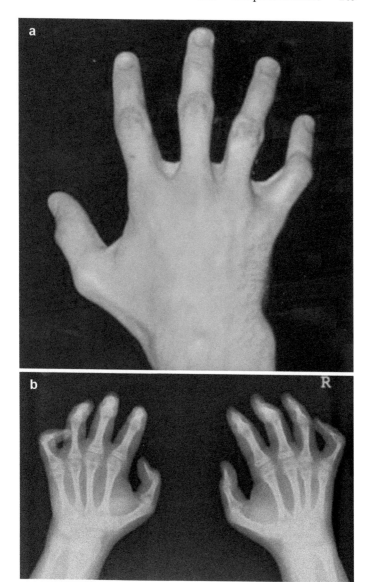

FIGURE 14.6 (**a**) Photograph of the right hand and (**b**) bilateral hand radiographs of a 14-year-old boy with CACP, showing (**a**) muscle wasting of the hand and contractures of the proximal interphalangeal joints, and (**b**) bilateral contractures of multiple digits with enlargement and mild flattening of the metacarpal epiphyses

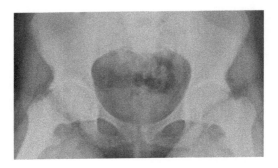

FIGURE 14.7 Frog-leg view of the pelvis of a 14-year-old boy with camptodactyly-arthropathy-coxa vara-pericarditis syndrome (CACP), showing extensive deformity of the hips with mushroom-shaped femoral heads, rounded proximal femoral physes, and acetabular dysplasia

References

1. Bonafe L, Cormier-Daire V, Hall C, et al. Nosology and classification of genetic skeletal disorders: 2015 revision. Am J Med Genet. 2015:167:2869–92.
2. Chalom EC, Ross J, Athreya BH. Syndromes and arthritis. Rheum Dis Clin N Am. 1997;23:709–27.
3. Cole WG, Makitie O. Primary disorders of connective tissue. In: Petty RE, Laxer RM, Lindsley CB, Wedderburn LR, editors. Textbook of Pediatric Rheumatology. 7th ed. Philadelphia: Elsevier; 2016. pp. 706–19.

Chapter 15
Benign and Malignant Tumors Involving the Musculoskeletal System

15.1 Introduction

Skeletal tumors can mimic arthritis and occasionally children are misdiagnosed and even treated for juvenile idiopathic arthritis (JIA) until the correct diagnosis is made.

Skeletal tumors can be differentiated into primary vs. metastatic/infiltrative, benign vs. malignant, by the bones involved – long bone vs. axial (vertebra, pelvis) vs. flat bones (ribs, clavicle), by location in the bone (epiphysis, metaphysis, diaphysis), and by age. Table 15.1 provides a list of the common skeletal tumors in children.

Tumors may present with asymptomatic swelling, pain, functional deficits secondary to local tumor spread, limp, pathologic fractures and/or constitutional features of systemic disease (fever, malaise, weight loss, etc.). Laboratory investigations include tests for acute phase reactants, CBC, biochemistry with LDH, uric acid, alkaline phosphatase and bone metabolism. Imaging tests include plain radiographs, technetium bone scan (most useful for osteoid osteoma, metastatic or infiltrative disease), CT and MRI [1]. Each imaging modality has advantages or limitations for various types of tumors and for investigating the extent and spread of the tumor. This chapter will discuss only the more common skeletal tumors a pediatrician is likely to face.

R.M. Laxer et al., *Pediatric Rheumatology in Clinical Practice*, 267
DOI 10.1007/978-3-319-13099-6_15,
© Springer-Verlag London 2016

TABLE 15.1 Common skeletal lesions and malignancies in children

Tumor	Type of tumor	Common age (years)	Common bones	Common location in bone	Source of tumor	Clinical presentation	Treatment
Osteoid osteoma	Primary benign	10–20	Femur, tibia, vertebra	Any	Osteogenic hamartoma	Pain, worse at night/rest	Excision/ablation, NSAIDs
Osteoblastoma	Primary benign[a]	>10	Vertebral arch		Bone	Pain	Resection, if possible
Osteosarcoma	Primary malignant	10–20	Femur, tibia, humerus	Metaphysis	Bone	Pain, swelling	Resection, amputation, chemotherapy
Osteochondroma	Primary benign[a]	5–15	Femur, tibia, humerus. rib	Metaphysis	Cartilage	Mass, local secondary changes > pain	Excision, if symptomatic
Chondroblastoma	Primary benign	10–20	Hip, shoulder, knee	Epiphysis	Cartilage	Pain, joint deformity	Excision, bone graft
Chondroma	Primary benign[a]	5–15	Hands, feet > humerus, femur	Tubular bone, metaphysis	Cartilage	Mass, pathologic fracture	Follow for changes, resection

Chondrosarcoma	Primary malignant	10–20	Rib, hand	Tubular bone, metaphysis	Cartilage	Swelling, pain	Resection, chemotherapy, irradiation
Giant cell tumor	Primary benign	10–20	Femur, radius		Stromal	Pain	Excision
Fibrous cortical defect	Primary benign	>2	Femur, tibia	Metaphysis	Fibrous	Incidental radiologic finding	None, unless >50 % of bone diameter
Unicameral bone cyst	Primary benign	6–10	Long bones	Metaphysis	Unclear	Localized swelling, pathologic fracture, pain	Curettage and insertion of bone chips
Aneurysmal bone cyst	Primary benign	10–20	Long bones	Metaphysis	Unclear	Pain, swelling	Curettage ± irradiation, sclerotherapy
Pigmented villonodular synovitis	Undefined	20–40, rare in children	Knee, ankle > hip	Joints, tendon sheath	Synovium vs. macrophage	Joint swelling, "bloody" aspiration	Excision for localized disease, intra-articular steroids, radiation for diffuse disease

(continued)

TABLE 15.1 (continued)

Tumor	Type of tumor	Common age (years)	Common bones	Common location in bone	Source of tumor	Clinical presentation	Treatment
Eosinophilic granuloma (isolated lesion)	Usually benign if isolated	5–10	Skull, spine, pelvis, femur	Diaphysis	Langerhans histiocytes	Pain, swelling	Curettage ± irradiation, corticosteroid injection
Ewing sarcoma	Primary Malignant	10–20	Femur, tibia, humerus, any bone	Diaphysis	Neuroectodermal	Pain, swelling, constitutional features	Resection, irradiation, chemotherapy
Leukemia	Infiltrative		Femur, tibia, radius	Metaphysis	Hematopoetic	Pain, constitutional features, purpura	Chemotherapy, bone marrow transplantation
Neuroblastoma	Metastasis	<5	Spine, skull, femur, rib, pelvis	Widespread	Neuroectodermal	Bone pain, constitutional features, arthritis	Chemotherapy, biologics

^aRare transformation to malignancy

15.2   Osteoid Osteoma

This tumor is a benign osteogenic hamartoma which causes symptoms by secreting prostaglandins. It usually presents in the second decade of life with severe pain, worse with rest, especially at night. The pain is highly responsive to NSAIDs or aspirin. Patients may develop a limp and secondary muscle atrophy and weakness near the affected site [1, 2]. The proximal femur is the most common site involved, followed by the proximal tibia and posterior aspects of the vertebra. Laboratory tests are normal and the tumor is detected by imaging. The classic radiologic appearance is of a dense nidus surrounded by a lucent ring which itself is surrounded by sclerotic bone (Fig. 15.1a). However, it may be difficult to observe the tumor on a plain radiograph. Since this tumor is metabolically active it is easy to detect these lesions by technetium bone scan. CT (more than MRI) is also useful in locating and diagnosing these lesions (Fig. 15.1b). Excision or radiofrequency ablation is curative, although there may be recurrences with the latter therapy. However, some patients may choose conservative treatment with NSAIDs since lesions often heal spontaneously or may be located in a region with high risk of surgical complications.

15.3   Osteochondroma

The most common benign childhood skeletal tumor is derived from cartilage origin. The tumor usually presents as an asymptomatic mass and is present in the metaphysis of long bones, often at the site of tendon insertions. The tumor extends as an exostosis from the bone and is capped by thick cartilage. Multiple exostoses can represent an autosomal dominant condition. Treatment is excision, if symptomatic (often causes nerve impingement) or growing rapidly. Malignant transformation may occur.

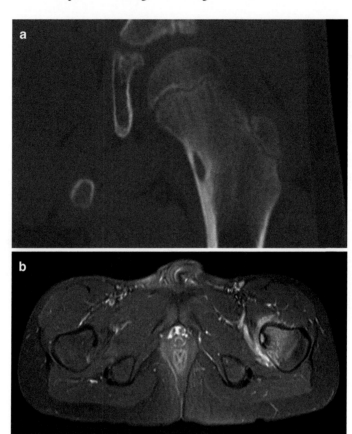

FIGURE 15.1 (**a**) Tomography of left proximal femur showing lucent bone lesion surrounded by sclerotic bone characterisitic of osteoid osteoma (Courtesy of Dr. Marilyn Ranson, The Hospital for Sick Children, Toronto, CA). (**b**) Transverse femur MRI showing more detail of this lesion with a dense nidus surrounded by a lucent ring which itself is surrounded by sclerotic bone and surrounding soft tissue edema (Courtesy of Dr. Marilyn Ranson, The Hospital for Sick Children, Toronto, CA)

15.4   Pigmented Villonodular Synovitis (PVNS)

It is unclear whether the source of this tumor is from synovium or secondary to inflammation/infection/recurrent trauma with the primary cell of macrophage source. This tumor is rare in childhood (most common between ages 20 and 40 years) and presents with painless joint swelling, often recurrent. The swelling has a boggy character and can be diffuse or localized to one part of the joint. It most commonly affects knees and ankles. Tendon sheaths may be affected. Aspiration of the joint reveals blood-stained, dark brown fluid. MRI findings of low density signal both on T1 and T2 images are suggestive of this tumor. There are two major types of PVNS: nodular or diffuse. It may be difficult to surgically treat diffuse PVNS and often anti-inflammatory treatment (mainly corticosteroid joint injection) and even local irradiation may be necessary.

15.5   Osteosarcoma

This is the most common malignant childhood primary skeletal tumor (~60 % of malignant bone tumors) and occurs primarily in the second decade of life. It is slightly more common in males and Caucasians. The tumor usually arises in the metaphysis of long bones, mainly the distal femur, proximal tibia and humerus [1, 3]. Occasionally there is a genetic etiology especially when associated with retinoblastoma and multiple exostoses. Prior radiation exposure is a risk factor.

Osteosarcoma usually presents with pain/limp and later swelling may be apparent. Alkaline phosphatase levels may be elevated. Osteosarcoma metastasizes early by hematogenous spread to the lungs and constitutional features of malaise, weight loss and even fever may be present. Clubbing may be a sign of spread to the lungs.

Radiographic findings are typical showing periosteal reaction (Codman's triangle) and a moth-eaten appearance with a soft tissue mass. Technetium bone scan shows increased uptake and CT/MRI are useful in delineating the extent of the disease which is diagnosed by a biopsy. Treatment includes surgery (amputation may be necessary) and chemotherapy which have improved the prognosis of this highly malignant tumor from a nearly 20 % to greater than 60 % 5 year survival rate, if non-metastatic. The extent and size of lung metastases determine the outcome of metastatic disease.

15.6   Ewing Sarcoma

This second most common childhood malignant skeletal tumor (10–15 %) is derived from primitive neural crest cell linage. It is more common in males and Caucasians, during the second decade of life. It can occur in any bone but is most common in the diaphysis of the long bones [1, 3]. The most common presentation is pain and swelling. However, Ewing sarcoma frequently presents with fever and increased acute phase reactants. The classic radiographic appearance is described as "onion-skin" or sunburst appearance surrounding a lytic lesion, which represents a large periosteal reaction. Pathologically sheets of small round cells are found, with positive staining for periodic acid-Schiff, often with chromosomal translocation. The tumor can metastasize to the lungs and other bones. Treatment includes surgical resection with irradiation and chemotherapy. Metastatic or proximal (e.g. pelvis) tumors carry a poor prognosis of 20–30 % 5-year survival rate.

15.7   Leukemia

This is by far the most common childhood malignancy to affect the skeleton. Nearly 30 % of leukemias present with skeletal pain and/or arthritis. The pain most commonly presents in the metaphyseal area near large joints, knees, ankles and wrists. It is important to suspect and correctly diagnose this disease as many patients have frank arthritis and some even have positive antinuclear antibodies and may be diagnosed with JIA. Blast cells may not be seen in peripheral smear until later in the disease. Premature administration of corticosteroids may mask the disease. There are several clinical and laboratory clues that can lead to the correct diagnosis (Table 15.2) [4, 5]. These include the timing and character of the pain, the degree of pain vs. physical findings, laboratory tests and imaging (Fig. 15.2). Bone marrow aspiration and biopsy are necessary for diagnosis.

TABLE 15.2 Clues for the diagnosis of leukemia vs. juvenile idiopathic arthritis (JIA) [4, 5]

Feature	Interpretation
Night pain	Uncommon in JIA
Location of pain	In leukemia bone pain is described
Pain vs. physical findings	In leukemia disproportionate pain vs. objective physical findings
Constitutional features	Can be present in both diseases but patients with leukemia appear more ill and wasted
CBC vs acute phase reactants	In leukemia discrepancy between highly elevated acute phase reactants and low (or even on the low side of normal) leukocytes and platelets
Biochemistry markers	In leukemia elevated lactate dehydrogenase and uric acid levels
Imaging	In leukemia metaphyseal rarefaction and marked periosteal reaction as well as increased uptake in multiple bones on technetium bone scan

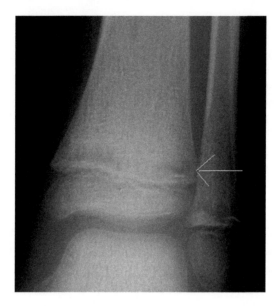

FIGURE 15.2 Metaphyseal rarefaction of distal tibia (*arrow*) as evidence of bone marrow infiltration in acute lymphoblastic leukemia (Courtesy of Dr. Marilyn Ranson, The Hospital for Sick Children)

15.8   Neuroblastoma

This neuroectodermal tumor of the sympathetic nervous system primarily affects children <5 years of age. Tumors metastasize early to the bone marrow and multiple bones and often present with bone pain and even arthritis. Patients usually have fever and increased acute phase reactants. This is the most common childhood tumor that metastasizes to bone. The spine, skull, femur and pelvis are affected most frequently. Radiographs show multiple lytic lesions and technetium bone scan shows increased uptake. PET-CT can be useful in identifying bone lesions.

References

1. Gereige R, Kumar M. Bone lesions: benign and malignant. Pediatr Rev. 2010;31:355–62.
2. Laurence N, Epelman M, Markowitz RI, et al. Osteoid osteomas: a pain in the night diagnosis. Pediatr Radiol. 2012;42:1490–501.
3. Arndt CA, Rose PS, Folpe AL, Laack NN. Common musculoskeletal tumors of childhood and adolescence. Mayo Clin Proc. 2012;87:475–87.
4. Jones OY, Spencer CH, Bowyer SL, et al. A multicenter case-control study on predictive factors distinguishing childhood leukemia from juvenile rheumatoid arthritis. Pediatrics. 2006;117:e840–4.
5. Zombori L, Kovacs G, Csoka M, Derfalvi B. Rheumatic symptoms in childhood leukaemia and lymphoma-a ten-year retrospective study. Pediatr Rheumatol Online J. 2013;11:20.

Index

R.M. Laxer et al., *Pediatric Rheumatology in Clinical Practice*,　279
DOI 10.1007/978-3-319-13099-6,
© Springer-Verlag London 2016

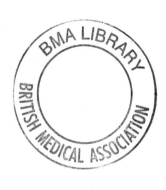

One

YOU SHOULDN'T TELL a story till it's over, and I'm not sure this one is. I'm not even certain when it really began, unless it was the morning Dad thrust my bawling brother Julius back in Mum's arms, and picked up the ringing telephone.

"The Palace? Why ever would they want me at the Palace?"

Anyone listening might have begun to think of royal garden parties, or something. But even back then, when I heard people saying things like 'the black horse' or 'the palace', I got a different picture. And that's because I've lived in hotels all my life. I don't even remember the first one, the Old Ship. Mum says it was small and ivy-covered, with only six bedrooms. Then Dad was manager of the North Bay. And later he was moved to the Queen's Arms, where we were living then.

"So what's the Palace's problem?"

He listened so long, and sighed so heavily, that Mum had looked up from trying to placate Julius with his favourite furry rabbit even before we heard Dad say,

"And I suppose you've forgotten I already have thirty beds to run here, not to mention a small son who makes sure nobody can even *think*."

That's when he noticed us watching, and, turning his back, finished almost in a whisper.

"All right. I'll drive over. Just to take a look."

I don't know what time he got back, but it was late. Our flat was above the kitchens, and the huge extractor fans had stopped humming. The only sounds left were the usual muffled telephones and scurrying footsteps.

At breakfast, he said to me:

"You ought to see it, Natalie. It's enormous. It's got over sixty bedrooms, and it sits on its lawns like a giant great wedding cake set out on a perfect green tablecloth."

"When can we come?"

He glanced at Mum, worn out from another bad night with Julius.

"Soon. Before I finish there. I'll take you over for the day."

But when we finally saw it, it wasn't for the day. It was with suitcases and boxes and bags.

"I'm sorry about this," Dad kept saying. "I really did think this was going to be a short job."

Mum tried to resettle Julius in the hot crush of his car seat. He squawked and struggled. And, tense from the packing, she complained the whole way.

"A few lumps of plaster falling in the guests' hair, you told me. Three weeks at most, till all the ceilings were fixed. And now it's wet rot. And dry rot. And problems with the piping, and the fire doors. Why can't the old manager cope? He's the one who let it all happen."

Dad knew there was no point in answering. He just drove.

"One man not up to his job," Mum grumbled. "And suddenly three weeks is three months, and Natalie has to come out of school a week before the holidays, and –"

We swung round the last bend, and she broke off. Before us stood the Palace, vast and imposing, silencing petty complaints.

Dad switched off the engine and Mum scrambled out. Julius immediately stopped struggling and fell quiet. Mum unstrapped him and lifted him into her arms. And as she carried him up the wide stone steps to the Palace, suddenly behind her the whole sky was ablaze. And on the lawns on either side of her, the peacocks spread their glimmering fans.

"See?" Dad whispered to me, triumphant. "A good omen!"

But I felt differently. I felt so strange. I think I must have been dizzy from the ride. I stumbled out of the car, and suddenly the sky seemed too high above me, the grass too green. And then one of the peacocks let out the most unholy cry, and I was filled with such unease.

Everyone thinks they can see things when they look back. It's nonsense, really, I expect.

Two

FORGET DAD COUNTING the bedrooms. The Palace had over a hundred rooms if, as well as the lounges and dining rooms and bars and verandahs, you counted hot attics and dark cellars. In less than a week, Dad had the last few stubborn guests shunted off. Then, within hours, some floors were taken up, some ceilings down, and I was living in a strange new world, peopled by men in overalls.

"Natalie, run up to the attics and tell Mr Forrester – he's the one with the beard – that some bloke's on the phone about his wallboard."

"Oh, no! The new sinks! Natalie, run round to the terrace and ask Ben if a couple of his lads can do a bit of unloading."

And off he'd stride, to sort out the plasterers, or make arrangements for work to start on yet another floor. Every so often he'd remember me, and the cry would go up.

"Where's Natalie? Anyone seen her?"

If nobody had, then he'd panic.

"Natalie! Can you hear me? Natalie!"

The shouts would echo through cavernous rooms and up lofty stairwells – "Natalie! *Natalie!*" – till one of the workmen spotted me arranging dusty glasses in rows, like soldiers, on the copper cocktail bar. Or cartwheeling across the empty ballroom. Or leaning over till my panties showed as I peered in cracked urns on the terrace.

"There she blows! Perfectly safe!"

I spent the summer skipping down corridors that had their carpets rolled, and holding endless imaginary conversations with the stone boy in the lily pond. For weeks, the Palace seemed more chaotic each time I picked my way down one of its great swooping staircases. Then, suddenly, the order was reversed. Day by day, dust sheets were whipped off tables and armchairs and sofas. Drills went back into toolchests. And cleaning began, till even my favourite gold cherubs over the mirrors glinted at me one morning, gleaming and bright.

Then, off to cadge a peppermint from one of the painters, I heard Dad taking a call.

"A south-facing double room. Yes, indeed. And dinner on both evenings. Thursday and Friday next."

I hurled myself at him, barely managing to keep quiet until he'd replaced the receiver.

"Is it opening again? Is that *it*? Are we *going*?"

Wincing, he reached down and lifted me onto the polished brown sea of the reception desk. He looked over his glasses at Mum, who'd been sorting out keys in the corner, and she sighed and gave a tired little nod.

"Natalie," he said gently. "I'm afraid we've got something rather awkward to tell you."

"Stay?" I said, wide-eyed, when I finally understood just what it was they were trying to explain. "Stay in the Palace for *ever*?"

They started to comfort me! How could they have known so little? How could they have got it so wrong? It had been my one dream all those long, long weeks. To stay! To somersault endlessly down the wide slopes of clover-studded lawn. Wander at will through drawing rooms, writing rooms, boathouses and conservatories. Bounce on the cherry-red sofas. Pick my way like a gymnast, toes pointed, arms outstretched, along the stone ledges of the terraces –

"Natalie?"

I stared at them.

"Natalie, sweet. You don't mind, do you? You won't pine for old friends? You will be all right?"

I nodded at them, dumb with joy.

Three

MUM HAD A hard time with the two of us when Julius was little. Even if my brother did ever finally fall asleep, Mum couldn't hide the fact that she was shattered.

"I'm sorry, Natalie," she'd say. "I know I promised. But I feel *sick* with tiredness. Can we do it another day?"

She'd give Dad one of her pleading looks, and, if he had the time, he'd take me off, across the lawns, through the rose garden, and then down the narrow twisty path that led through the dark belt of trees. It almost hurt to step out again, into the brightness of the open field. And that's where we first met Tulip, still as a statue in the sea of corn.

"Is that a scarecrow?"

Dad peered against the sudden glare.

"No. I do believe that it's a little girl."

"What is she doing out here, all alone?"

Dad shrugged.

"We'll ask." He took my hand and called across. "He-llooo! He-llooo!"

She turned to face us, and I could see that she was nursing something.

"Is that a *kitten*?"

I was off in an instant. The Palace had stuffy old cats. But a kitten! Bliss! Dad roared after me. "Natalie! Think of the crop!" And I came to a halt. Even I realised the farmers were our neighbours, and must be friends. So I stood, burning with impatience, while this stranger my age stepped carefully towards us, spreading the corn with her free hand and picking her way so gently that by the time she reached us I couldn't see a sign of the track she had taken.

The kitten's eyes weren't even open yet.

"What's its name? What are you going to call it?"

Dad touched my shoulder.

"It would be more polite, Natalie, to ask the young lady her name first."

He looked at her expectantly. But she just tossed her unbrushed hair out of her eyes and stared as if he'd dropped from outer space.

Dad tried again.

"This," he said, patting me, "this is Natalie. And I am Mr Barnes, from the hotel."

Again we waited. And then, finally:

"Tulip," she said.

I couldn't believe that was her name. I thought she must mean the kitten. And sometimes I wonder if that's the reason I dropped everything to run across and say hello to her a few days later, when she appeared at the edge of the playground. Because, still almost a stranger in my new school, I couldn't miss the chance to say something so silly and bold.

"Hello, Tulip!"

She stared at me, and I faltered. The silence between us grew. And then, too embarrassed to come to my senses, I added the really stupid bit.

"Do you want to be friends?"

Four

I PAID FOR the privilege (if privilege is what it was). Nobody else would have Tulip in their gang. They knew from experience that she was out of school more often than in. (That's why I'd never seen her.) From that day on, I spent countless hours scuffing alone round the playground, desperately hoping that she'd show up, or that some soft soul in one of the busy swarms of children whooping round me would crack and say the words I longed to hear.

"Forget silly old Tulip. She's never here, anyway. Come and play with us."

I look back and think I must have been mad. What sort of friendship is it when one of the pair is hardly ever there, and the other is never permitted to go off and find her?

On this, my father was adamant.

"I'm not even discussing it, Natalie. You are not

going over to Tulip's house. She can come here as often as she likes. But you're not going there. And that is final."

Why was he so firm about it? What had he seen that first day that made him so convinced the Pierces' farm was no place for a daughter of his? Most run-down smallholdings are ringed with disembowelled machinery. Most small-time farmers keep frustrated dogs chained up to bark at every passing sparrow. And we didn't meet Tulip's parents. For all Dad knocked and knocked, no one appeared.

A dozen times a week I'd say to him:

"Let's go back and try again. I haven't seen her for days. I probably won't see her again, *ever*, at this rate, if I can't go and find her."

"No."

"Maybe she's ill."

"I doubt it, Natalie."

"It's not her fault her parents don't think school's important."

"If I were you, I'd make some other friends. Because nothing's going to change here. You are not going to be allowed to go to Tulip's house. And that is that."

Was I just being stubborn? What sort of magic did

she have for me? All I know is I never made the effort to find another friend. I didn't even put myself out to steal enough good things from the kitchens to wheedle my way into one of the school gangs. Instead, I stayed aloof; and during evenings and weekends I floated round the Palace, presumably content with the glancing interest of bored guests, and my own company, till I'd see her standing on the edge of the lawns.

Then my heart leapt up, and across I'd fly.

"Tulip! Where have you *been*? It's been *ages*. What do you want to *do*?"

Five

WE DID EVERYTHING. We went everywhere. We were called in from lawns and potting sheds, shrubberies and terrace gardens. When the cold weather came, they'd look for us in lounges and coffee rooms, alcoves and blanket stores. Sometimes it was awkward to come out because, for the last hour, we'd been wrapped in the folds of the plush ruby curtains, eavesdropping on some unwitting pair of bickering guests. But mostly we'd appear soon after we heard the determined footsteps and the call.

"Time to go home now, Tulip."

"Can't I stay?"

"Your parents will worry."

It wasn't true. If Tulip's parents worried, they'd have shown up a dozen times before, when no one had even realised she was still with me till I was ordered off to bed. But Dad would keep a straight face. So would she.

"Can I come back tomorrow?"

"If you like."

Maybe she would. Maybe she wouldn't. (I'd be waiting, whichever.) Sometimes Dad would notice me drifting round in a trance of solitude, and, realising how busy he'd been lately, offer to take me fishing. We'd set off in the quiet hour after lunch, and there she'd be, hanging around the field end of the walk through the spinney.

"You can send her home if you like," I'd say softly, stung that she hadn't bothered to show up for me.

But he'd greet her as cheerfully as usual.

"Coming along?"

She was no good at fishing. (Dad said that everything swam off the minute it saw her shadow.) He'd catch one thing after another, I'd do all right, and she'd get nothing. But she seemed happy enough. And so did he. He never seemed bored on the afternoons Tulip came.

"What was that game you two were playing yesterday, when Mrs Scott-Henderson complained about the noise?"

"*Rats in a Firestorm*."

"Did you find somewhere more sensible to play it?"

She grinned.

"We moved down to the cellars, and called it *Hogs in a Tunnel*, instead."

He shook his head.

"Very pleasant. Though I suppose it's still less of a bother than that game you were playing all last week."

"Which? *Fat in the Fire*?"

"It was *Malaria!* most of last week," I reminded her.

"Why can't you invent some quiet ones?"

"I don't invent them," I told him. "Tulip invents the games."

He turned towards her.

"So," he said. "How about it, Tulip?"

She cocked her head to one side. "There's *Road of Bones*. That's very quiet. And we play *Days of Dumbness* quite a lot. No noise at all in that one."

He shuddered. "*Days of Dumbness!* *Road of Bones!* Don't the two of you ever play anything pleasant?"

She was grinning again now.

"I suppose you played things like *Happy Families* and *Tickle the Baby* when you were young."

"Yes," he said. "That's the sort of thing we used to play back in the good old days."

She gave him her flirty look.

"What's the worst thing you ever did, Mr Barnes?"

"When I was a child?"

She nodded.

If I'd asked him that question, he'd never have given a sensible answer. But Tulip could make Dad talk about anything, anything at all, and so he fell quiet, thinking.

"The thing I feel worst about, even after all this time, is dropping my grandfather's tortoise on the garden path," he told us finally. "I didn't have the guts to go and tell, so I just shoved it out of sight under the nearest bush."

He still looked uneasy, remembering.

"How old were you?" I asked.

"Eight." He made a quick calculation. "Twenty-seven years ago!"

"Did it smash?" Tulip demanded.

The word she chose repelled him, you could tell. He picked a different one with care.

"Its shell did crack, yes."

"Was it an accident?"

"Of course it was an accident," he said sharply. "You don't suppose I *threw* it?"

"No," she said hastily.

There was a silence. Then Tulip said:

"You should have put it in the freezer to kill it."

Dad's face was a picture.

"It's the kindest way, for fish and terrapins," she assured him. "Probably for tortoises, as well."

He'd forgotten his fishing line. He was staring at her now.

"Tulip, how would you ever know that?"

"I suppose I just heard it somewhere. And remembered it."

Dad turned to me.

"Did you know?"

I wanted so much to say I did. But Tulip would have known I was fibbing.

"No," I said sullenly.

He turned back to her.

"And do the things you hear worry you?"

"No," she said. "Sometimes I think about them for a bit. But mostly I'm interested more than I'm worried."

There was a flurry underneath her float.

"Is that a bite?" he asked, happy to be distracted. "Have you been lucky for once? Is that a bite?"

"No," she said, not even looking. "No, it's not."

Six

I DID GO to her house, of course. But only once. I can't remember what fired me up. Had I, for once, something to tell her that I should be brave enough to sidle to the edge of the lawn, then so casually slip out of sight in the shadows? Those huge, overhanging trees must have given a sense of foreboding to the venture. But I didn't falter, and, out in the sunlight again, stayed on the far side of the fence till I was beyond the view from the highest Palace window. Hotels are filled with bored people. You can always be sure that, whatever you are doing, there will always be somebody standing and watching.

I hated Tulip's house. It wasn't just that the carpets were stained and the furniture battered. It was that Tulip herself seemed different, just a shell, as if she had slipped away invisibly and left some strange, strained imitation in her place to say to me, "What shall we do now?" or, "Want another biscuit?"

I pushed the packet of damp crumbs aside. I'd have suggested going into her bedroom, but the glimpse of a stained sheet spread over a chair to dry as she kicked closed the door had warned me that wouldn't be welcome.

"Shall we go in the yard?"

I wanted to get out of the kitchen. Tulip's mother was giving me the creeps with her beg-pardon smile and her tireless, tuneless humming; as if, in that horrible, smelly, sunless back room, she'd completely forgotten a song was supposed to have a melody, let alone a beginning and ending. Hearing that awful, interminable drone was like listening to a robot pretend to be a person.

The back yard had clumps of weeds waist high. But there were far too many smashed bottles lying about for us to play most of our creeping games. So, in desperation, I said:

"Let's go and find your kitten."

She looked at me blankly.

"Well," I corrected myself, feeling stupid. "Cat, by now."

"We don't have a cat."

"You were carrying one the day I met you."

Her eyes went pebble hard.

"I expect I had to give it away."

I knew she was lying. So, in my eyes, of course, it was a merciless cat killer I met when, retreating from the unpromising yard, we came face to face with Mr Pierce, striding in through another door. I watched as he filled a cracked cup with water, drank it down, refilled it, drank more, then turned back from the sink. His eyes came to rest on me, and never moved till I snatched up my jacket and, burbling excuses, rushed away.

"I'm sorry I had to go like that," I said to her next morning at school. "I suddenly remembered I was supposed to –"

And off I went again. Burble-burble. Burble-burble. Tulip looked cross and bored until I stopped. Then she said:

"Dad's all right when you're used to him."

But I had no intention of giving him even one more try. From that day on, I stopped nagging Dad about letting me go there, and used the excuse he had taught me to save Tulip's feelings,

"They won't let me near dogs like Elsa."

And stayed away.

Seven

AND I SAW lots of her at school. She had no other friends. Nobody else could stand the embarrassment of pretending that they believed her awful lies.

"The army's borrowing one of our fields today. When I get home, they're going to let me drive a tank."

"Oh, I really believe that, Tulip!"

"So likely!"

They'd walk off, scoffing. I'd stare at the ground, and, guess what, I'd feel *sorry* for her. I knew she was making a fool of me in front of everyone. (Only an idiot would make a show of believing her rubbish.) But instead of just walking away, exasperated, like everyone else, I'd try taking her arm and distracting her.

"Want to play *Road of Bones* on the way home?"

She'd shake me off, rude and ungrateful. Even back then I had to ask myself why I stayed around. It wasn't out of pity, I knew that. Nobody *has* to carry on telling ridiculous lies, even after it's obvious that no one believes them.

"I've won a big competition. I found a scratchcard in my cornflakes and I was lucky. So now I've won this beautiful yellow silk dress."

Next time we bought sweets in Harry's supermarket, I'd linger by the breakfast cereal shelves.

"There's nothing about a competition on any of these packets."

"No. It was a scratchcard inside."

"Strange that no one else got one."

"They only sent out a few as a special anniversary thing. That's why the prize is a yellow silk dress. It's the very same one that the model wore in their first advert."

That's what Dad came to call the Tulip touch – that tiny detail that almost made you wonder if she might, just for once, be telling the truth.

"And then this man went grey and keeled over. And as I was phoning for the ambulance, his fingers kept twitching, and his wedding ring made a tiny little pinging noise against the metal of the drain."

"So I wasn't at school because the police needed one extra person my age and size, for a line-up. They wouldn't say why they'd arrested the girl, but one of them did tell me that he thought she was Polish."

"Ah!" Dad would murmur in unfeigned admiration. "Polish? The perfect Tulip touch!"

She'd give him a pained wooden stare. "Sorry?"

"Nothing."

He'd turn away, of course, to hide his grin. But I'd be left to see the look of venom on her face. Tulip loathed being teased. It was as if the moment these stupid stories were out of her mouth, she believed them completely, and anyone who queried even a tiny part of them was going to be her enemy, and hated for ever.

So it was Dad, not me, who risked a bit of mischief a couple of weeks later.

"So where's the great yellow dress, Tulip? How come you haven't brought it round to show us yet?"

She looked surprised. "Didn't I tell you? I had it ready in a bag. Then Mum knocked over a bottle of bleach, and some got on the sleeve. So she's posted it off to a big firm in Chichester that does a lot of mending for the royal family, to see if they can patch it from the hem."

Dad watched her, spellbound. Once she was gone, he turned to Mum.

"Poor little imp. What sort of squashing must she get at home, to think she has to make up all this stuff to impress us?"

Mum just said irritably:

"You'd think she had more than enough brains to know better!"

And you would, too. She was miles cleverer than me. If it weren't for her missed days, and undone homework, she would have beaten me in every test. But, even in good weeks, Miss Henson had problems with Tulip.

"Please try and settle down. You're distracting everybody round you."

"Now that's not what I told you to do, is it?"

"Tulip! I warn you, I have had *enough*!"

If she'd spoken to me that sharply, I'd have died of fright. But Tulip didn't care. A moment later, she'd be rushing out of her seat across the room.

"I can see Julia's rubber on the floor!"

And a minute or so later:

"Now I'm going across to help Jennifer with her project."

There was a plaintive and immediate wail.

"Stop her, Miss Henson! I don't want her help!"

Out came the tongue. (Tulip's, not Jennifer's.)

"Tulip! Back to your table! Sit down! And stop being such a nuisance!"

I sat so quiet I was hardly there. That's why she left us side by side, I expect. So I could water Tulip's fidgets down. But somehow we went together well, and things worked out. We were the triangles in primary band. We shared counting the lunch money two months in a row (though, now I look back, I realise that was probably Miss Henson's way of getting the job done properly through Tulip's month of office). And we were the Ugly Sisters in the Christmas play.

At first, I could tell, both Miss Henson and Mr Barraclough were deeply dubious about giving Tulip the part she begged for so piteously.

"I have to warn you, Tulip. If you miss more than a couple of rehearsals, we'll have to take the part off you. So are you sure?"

She nodded vigorously.

"And I must have a note from your father saying he won't mind you coming in for the evening performances."

Tulip's keen look turned sour.

"Nobody else has to bring in any note."

Miss Henson sighed.

"I'm sorry, Tulip. It's just that Mr Barraclough hasn't forgotten yet."

When she'd walked off, I asked Tulip:

"Hasn't forgotten what?"

"Last time. Before you came. I was a Dancing Bean."

"Was it difficult?"

(It seemed the best way of asking, 'What went wrong?')

"I did it fine," she said. "I learned the song. I knew the dance. But then something came up. So I couldn't do it."

I'd been fobbed off with that 'something came up' too often myself. But in the first flush of being her Ugly Sister, I felt generous.

"You'd think he'd *want* you to have a good part this time."

She executed what I could only take to be a short snatch of Bean Dance.

31

"It wouldn't have mattered so much, except for the others."

"Others?"

"The other beans. The dance was a bit complicated, you see. So they couldn't do it without me."

"Oh."

I had a sudden vision of everyone trying to get through the big night with only one Ugly Sister. Me. But, in the end, there wasn't any trouble. Her mother sent in the note. Tulip showed up every day that we had a rehearsal. And she and I turned out to be the stars of the show. Tulip's witchy foot-stamping frenzies and my vacuous no-one-at-home stare were far more fun to watch than prissy Cinderella's tears. Each time we stumbled off stage, Mr Barraclough was waiting with the grease stick. My first few discreet spots grew, scene by scene, into a riot of measles. He'd spray more cobwebs onto Tulip's frizzy green wig, and push us both on again, hissing,

"Brilliant, the pair of you! Keep it up!"

And so we did, three evenings in a row, getting the loudest laughter all the way through, and the longest applause at the end. After the last show I was so forlorn I refused to let anyone take off my make-up. The giant spots rubbed off on my pillowcase, and Tulip had to hand in her green wig in the morning. But no one could wipe the performance out of us.

"Will you two stop lolling against one another! If you don't, I shall separate you."

"Natalie, don't nudge Tulip when you know the answer yourself. You're not a dummy. Put up your own hand, please."

"Tulip, she's not a puppet on a string. Just because you need to go, it doesn't follow that Natalie has to go with you."

Halfway through January, Miss Henson finally moved us apart. We wailed and fussed.

"It isn't fair! We weren't being naughty. We were just being *sisters*, like in the play."

"Hard cheese," she said brutally. "I'm afraid that was *last* year."

And that, of course, set off the next game. *That Was Last Year.* The silliest remark would set it off.

"Marcie can't find her gloves."

"No. That was last year. She's looking for her panties now."

"Have you seen Miss Henson's new car?"

"That was last year. She came on a broomstick this morning."

33

They were so stupid and unfunny, we only whispered them. But still they sent us into such spasms of amusement that the others would gather round us in the playground.

"What's the big joke?"

"Nothing."

We'd stick our knuckles in our mouths and snigger some more.

"Oh, leave them. They're just being silly."

And so we were. So silly that, before I realised what was happening, the taint of unpopularity had thickened and spread.

"Oh, *please* don't make me sit by Natalie. She just giggles all the time, and makes faces with Tulip."

"I'm not sitting with her, either!"

Miss Henson caught the flu. Her father had to go to hospital. And everyone she tried to seat us beside put up a really hard fight. It's strange to think that we go down whole different paths because of accidents in other people's lives. My friendship with Tulip could have been derailed, or, at the very least, diluted a little.

But flu. A broken hip. A bit of squawking round the class.

And she gave up.

"All right, then. If you promise to behave your-selves, I'll give you one more chance. Just one."

Eight

WHAT WERE WE like then, the pair of us, Tulip and Natalie? I lift a photograph out of the box, and see us laughing. We look happy enough. But do old photos tell the truth? "Smile!" someone orders you. "I'm not wasting precious film on sour faces." And so you smile. But what's behind? You take the one Dad snapped by accident when Tulip came down the cellar steps just as he was fiddling in the dark with his camera. Suddenly the flash went off, and he caught her perfectly (if you don't count the rabbity pink eyes). She's a shadow in the arched entrance of that dark tunnel. And how does she look in that, the only one to be taken when no one was watching?

Wary, would you say? Or something even stronger? One look at that pale and apprehensive face, and you might even think *haunted*. But there's something else that springs to mind. I turn the photo in my hand, and try to push the word away. But it comes back at me, time and again. I can't get rid of it. If you didn't know her better, you'd have said she looked *desolate*.

And yet Tulip loved the Palace. Every inch of it. I'd watch her endlessly running her fingertips along the swirling banisters and gritty stone ledges and dimpled bar tops as if, by sheer touching, she could make the whole place hers.

"Natalie, you're so *lucky*."

I'd shrug. I knew it, but it seemed rude to agree; as if, in admitting it, I'd be halfway to saying that I would have gladly died a thousand deaths rather than swap my life with hers. And these days Tulip rarely hung around the cornfields. She came as often as she could, sucking up to Mum, flirting with Dad.

"Good morning, Mr Barnes."

"Morning, Tulip, my flower. But I do have to warn you that no one gets late breakfast in this hotel, even here in the kitchens, without first settling with the Manager."

"What's the price today?"

"Let me see . . . It's Saturday, isn't it? And High Season. So I'm afraid it's going to be – a hug and three kisses."

He'd take off his glasses and she'd count the kisses out onto his cheek.

"One. Two. Three. And the hug. There!"

"Right," he'd say. "Now that you've paid, you must have another sausage."

He'd flip it on her plate, his party trick. But she'd be watching, not the arc it was making through the air, but the sausage itself. For Tulip loved the food. I was forever losing sight of her for a few minutes, only to find her in the kitchens, her mouth stuffed with something she'd already begged, staring at treats to come: the creamy trifles and the chocolate roulades; the cherry meringue pies she loved above all else.

"Want to come up to the toy room?"

"In a bit."

A few minutes later, she'd trail up the last of the steep wooden stairs and join me, rooting through drifts of abandoned games and toys. The sort of people who bring children to the Palace have never been the types to go scouring the grounds on their last day for lost rounders bats and mislaid dolls. So if we were bored with hurling hard apples at the stone boy in the lily pond, or racing up and down the gravel paths, then we'd go up and find something different in the toy room. We had a craze on the pogo stick, and learned to fly the battered kites. Tulip mastered the fretwork saw, and we even had short passions for the faded old sewing cards and the prissy little flower press.

"What do you think? Dress-ups?"

The trunks were brilliant, spilling with feather boas, and muffs, and tunics with military frogging.

"Do you suppose the people who owned all these really old things are *dead*?"

I held my favourite taffeta frock against me.

"They must be. Most things get sent on now. Dad says he spends most of Tuesday posting packages to careless people."

She jammed a brown felt hat down hard on my head.

"Now you're Miss Henson's mother."

I threw a velvet cape around her shoulders and handed her a tattered parasol.

"And you're Mr Barraclough's great aunt."

We minced round the attics in our ill-fitting high heels.

"Did you see my nephew's splendid recent production of *Cinderella*?"

"Indeed I did."

"And did you notice those two astonishingly

talented young actresses, Tulip and Natalie? I thought that Tulip was by far the best."

"I preferred Natalie."

"No. Tulip."

"Natalie."

"Tulip."

We fell, wrestling, onto the heaps of old clothes. My nose filled with the stink of mothballs.

"Even-stevens?" I panted.

She let go of me.

"Even-stevens."

The hours spun past. Time had two speeds for me. The racing kaleidoscopic tumble of days spent with Tulip, when the first of the peacocks' bloodcurdling evening shrieks made me look at my watch with astonishment. And then the endless drag of days alone, when only a few miserable minutes crawled by between each desperate inspection of the clock.

There was scant sympathy at hand.

"If you're bored, play with Julius."

"I'm not bored."

I was, though. Not bored enough to play with my brother, but bored enough to feel that every minute spent away from Tulip was not real living, just a waiting time.

"Well, play with Julius anyway."

And so I did. Sometimes with good grace, sometimes with bad. But always feeling there was something missing, and that the real day I should be having was taking place somewhere half a dozen fields away, beyond the spinney.

With Tulip.

Nine

S HE BOUGHT JULIUS a plastic toad for his birthday. We stood in front of it in the charity shop.

"It's a bit scratched," she worried.

"He won't mind that. He probably won't even notice."

"You don't think he'd prefer something furry?"

"No. I think he'll like this."

Like it? He fell in love. He instantly named it Mr Haroun (after a recent guest who'd spoiled him rotten) and carried it round all day. At bathtime it disappeared under a towel, and when one of the Austrian ladies staying a week had to wait twenty minutes for a drink because half the hotel staff were searching for the toad, she persuaded her sister to lay aside the rose tapestry she was working on, and run up a sort of baby back-pack that kept Mr Haroun safe, but left Julius's hands free. Julius's loyalties were fierce. The Austrian guests moved on (though not before appliquéing Mr Haroun's name in glossy silk letters on the tie-down flap). And Tulip reaped all the credit. Everyone who passed through the Palace admired the way the backpack was designed to keep the toad safe, but let him see and breathe. And, if we were around, Julius inevitably pointed to Tulip and said proudly:

"She gave it me."

Guests would fall over themselves to congratulate Tulip. They admired everything about the backpack: its design, the silk lettering, the beautiful stitching. Tulip soaked up the praise, grinning modestly and flapping her hands in an embarrassed fashion. It never bothered Julius that Tulip was accepting compliments for someone else's work. Why should it? To him, only his precious toad mattered, and Tulip had definitely given him that. But what is strange is that it never bothered me. Guests would lean forward on sofas to flatter Tulip, and their companions would turn aside and tap me on the arm.

"Now, *isn't* your friend clever?"

And so in thrall to Tulip that everything she did was fine by me, I'd feel as proud of her as if she could sew.

Ten

ONE OF MY jobs was taking Julius to nursery on my way to school. Down the drive, over the bridge (walking on the side with the *pavement*) and up the path to the porch, where all the others were struggling to get out of their brightly coloured wellies and raincoats.

For a goodbye, Julius would lift his face and purse his lips to give me a giant smacker.

"Kissypots!"

He'd turned from a sleepless monster into an easy and affectionate child. "Devil to angel" said my parents. And even I enjoyed his constant stream of bright prattle as we strolled along together, hand in hand. I'd been forbidden to make arrangements to meet Tulip on school mornings because I'd been late so often on days when she didn't show. But, as often as not, out she'd jump from behind someone's front wall, or one of the pillars of the bridge, startling me every time.

She'd fall in step.

"Want to play *Stinking Mackerel*?"

"All the way? Even the people at the bus stop?"

"All the way. Everyone. Even Mrs Bodell."

So everyone who passed got enough of the game to unnerve them. We weren't *rude*, exactly. It was all done with a wrinkle of the nose, a tiny sniff, maybe even a fleeting look of disgust. Some days, with everyone bent double against the wind, it didn't work. On others, we must have left a trail of worried people. Often we'd turn and catch them plucking at their clothes, trying to look as if they were simply pulling a jacket straight, or tightening a belt, when we knew they were anxiously checking for odours.

Mrs Bodell, though, rumbled us thoroughly. She took no cheek, and some of her threats were awesome.

"I'm catching the bus into Urlingham now. But as soon as I get back I shall speak to your head teacher. Don't think I don't know your parents, Natalie Barnes. *And* how ashamed they'll be to hear of your behaviour."

So we'd do Mrs Bodell. But only half-heartedly, safe behind her giant rump. And even then I'd cheat,

45

unwrapping my lunch bag as I walked by the stop, and lowering my nose to it as though to imply that all the sniffing and nose-wrinkling was nothing to do with her, but because of my sandwich.

Safe in the playground, I'd start to moan at Tulip.

"You're ruder than I am. How come it's always *my* name she broadcasts to the world?"

But I knew the answer, anyway. Mum wasn't the first to point out that games with Tulip had a habit of starting well for two, and ending badly for one. I was the usual victim. But once or twice she tried her luck with Julius. I called a halt to *Putting On The Bag*. But then she started something called *Babe in the Wood*. One after another, while we were walking him, we'd vanish into the trees. Soon he'd be fretting. Then I'd materialise as calmly as if I'd never been gone. He'd spin round, and there was Tulip, back without a word. Somehow she'd distract him, and I'd be gone again. He'd turn, upset and confused, to find that Tulip had disappeared as well. The game used to drive him wild with fear and rage. And why are my memories of it so strong, unless we played it for weeks? Maybe we only stopped because Mum caught us at it. She heard the screams, and running up, found Julius with tears spurting from his eyes, spitting a blaze of gibberish.

"Out here, right now! Both of you!"

I stepped out at once. But this time Tulip had vanished for good and proper. That didn't bother Mum. She raised her voice and warned her anyway.

"You listen to me, Tulip Pierce! If I ever catch you tormenting Julius again, you'll be in trouble! And, as for you, Natalie!"

As for me, I was sent upstairs earlier than Julius for a whole week. Whichever of them it was, Mum or Dad, deliberately called out "Bedtime, now, Natalie!" in front of the guests, who looked up in astonishment from their first gins and tonics. You could almost hear them whispering to one another: "Bedtime? Surely the child must be ten years old, at least!" From that day on, I wouldn't join in games with Julius unless he quite enjoyed them. But Tulip didn't mind because, what with Christmas coming up, she was happy to be on her very best behaviour. Tulip *loved* Christmas at the Palace. At her house, we knew, the decorations amounted to little more than a set of chipped Nativity figures and some wobbly-headed Santa she never properly described. The wrappings for her presents were ironed over from last year. And the only special foods were the turkey and Christmas pudding.

Still, Tulip's pleading made my parents uneasy at first.

"Can I come early? For breakfast?"

"But, Tulip, won't your parents mind? Won't they want you at home with them?"

Tulip put on her false face.

"Oh, no. They don't mind. They say it's just a shame I don't have any brothers or sisters to share the day, and if I want to be with Natalie, they're happy for me."

It didn't sound all that likely. But Mum allowed herself to be convinced.

"In that case, I'm sure we'd be delighted to have you."

I look back now, and wonder what price Tulip paid for Christmas at the Palace. More than the other guests, I'll bet. I knew that even back then. For once, as we were strolling home together after school, I heard a vicious bellow, and looked up to see Mr Pierce leaning out of his truck window.

"Better get home before me, Tulip, or I'll snatch you bald-headed!"

I stood, rigid. Snatch her *bald-headed*? But Tulip had already fled. I followed her as far as the corner, picking up things that spilled out of her schoolbag, and thinking about the odd things I'd heard her saying in our games. "I'll peel you alive, like a banana!" "Smile at me wrong today, and I'll crush you!" "I'll make your eyes look like slits in a grapefruit!" I'd always put them down to Tulip being clever – good with words. But was I wrong? Was it Tulip I'd been hearing, or her terrifying father?

No Christmas on earth would have been worth it for me. But I'd been spoiled. As long as I could remember, every December had blazed scarlet and gold. Bright coloured lanterns winked along the terraces. There were at least five decorated trees. Everything glittered and sparkled, and the food was amazing.

"Can we have pies with battlements?"

"Natalie, when did we ever *not* have pies with battlements at Christmas?"

"And will there be some of those great long pink fishes on a dish?"

"Salmon, Tulip. Yes, there'll be salmon."

"And wine jellies, like last year?"

"Yes. Wine jellies."

"And can I turn on the blinking lights?"

Dad grinned.

"Yes, Tulip. You can turn on the blinking lights."

We all indulged her at Christmas. It was, my father

said wryly, the only time Tulip ever acted her age. Her eyes kept widening. Her mouth kept falling open. And once, like Julius, she was even found scrabbling under the tree, shaking all the empty wrapped boxes, just to be sure that what she'd been told was true, and they were really only there for show.

Each year, Mum found some way to smarten her up a bit.

"Here, Tulip. This dress belongs to Mrs Stoddart's Cecily. But she's wearing her green one, and we think this will fit you. It's just for today, mind. You mustn't run off with it."

There was a sticky moment, but Dad managed to save it.

"And Mrs Stoddart mustn't run off with you!"

So Tulip pretended that she hadn't heard, or didn't mind, and let herself slip into enchantment. She cuddled the frock till Mum pushed her into the office. There, Tulip raised her arms and Mum lifted off her thin, mock-crochet top, and unhooked her cheap skirt. The deep blue velvet of the frock tumbled all over her, falling in folds that turned her spindly thinness into height, and hid her battered shoes.

"And can I wear it all day?"

"All day."

And all day we caught her stroking invisible puckers and creases out of the velvet, and seeking out mirrors. Time and again she'd think of clever ways of getting rid of me for a few minutes. And when I rushed back, she'd be smiling at herself in the glass as she watched the reflection of her solitary make-believe dance swirls and curtsies.

Dad kept creeping up on her from the sides.

"Unbutton your beak, Tulip."

Her eyes closed. A blissful look stole over her face as she opened her mouth as wide as a young thrush.

He popped in the canapé, or vol-au-vent, or whatever. She learned the hard way about spoiling her appetite for lunch. And when, after dinner, it was clear she'd given no thought at all to getting home, Dad pulled her aside for a moment.

"Tulip, aren't you going to get into hot water if you're late?"

On went the false face.

"They know I'm probably going to stay the night. They said I could."

His troubled eyes met hers. He looked down first.

"All right, then. If you're *sure*."

And he took Tulip by one hand and me by the other, and with Julius leading the way on his brand new tricycle (indoors for one day only, all guests warned), he marched us towards the piano. I expect we were dreadful at singing. But they would have drowned us out, that strange and hearty assortment of people who choose to spend Christmas in a big hotel. Some patted our shoulders and pointed to the place on the carol sheet. And others, who had no idea how much we'd already eaten, slipped unwrapped sweets into our hands. I remember the blue-rinsed ladies had gold teeth that winked in the candlelight. And the men often stank of tobacco. Mr Hearn's hands swept effortlessly up and down the keys. And if you looked sideways at Tulip in her beautiful blue dress, chirruping out *Good King Wenceslas* and *Silent Night*, her face radiant, you would never have thought that she'd have to go home, and face a very different, more ugly, sort of music in the morning.

Eleven

NOT THAT SHE couldn't hand it out herself. Dad said it first.

"I reckon some mean thoughts go on behind those pretty smiles of hers."

And he was right. On our first day back at school after the holidays, Tulip was waiting for me at the gate.

"You've got it, haven't you? You didn't forget?"

I handed it over. Her eyes sparkled, and she went dancing off in search of Jamie Whitton. She thrust the little box into his hand.

"What's this?"

"What does it look like? It's a Christmas present."

He shook it suspiciously. "It's a bit late for that."

If she'd said anything, he would have been even more wary. But she just shrugged. She had a gift for making people believe her.

He glanced round. Miss Henson was standing on the steps. The bell would go any minute.

"Why did you get me a present?"

"I just did."

"I didn't get you one."

"That's all right."

She managed to look both shy and careless at the same time. I knew then it was going to work.

"Tulip –"

"Shh!" she said to me sharply. And then, to Jamie: "Go on, then. Open it. It won't bite you."

I could have said, "No, don't. It's not a real present. Just something stupid we did yesterday." Then Jamie would have stuffed it back at her, and she'd have dropped it. And then, of course, she would have walked away. From him. From me.

So I stood and watched as he tugged gingerly at the knotted silver thread, and unwrapped the glistening paper. He tipped the lid back. The little black curls of dried dog mess sat in their crumpled tissue nest.

"Happy Christmas!" crowed Tulip.

"Happy Christmas!" I echoed.

Bravely, he tried to defend himself. "It isn't Christmas any more. And so the joke's on you."

And probably just about anyone else in the class could have carried it off. But not Jamie. Tulip knew how to choose her victims. From the moment she'd spotted the little desiccated pile beside the radiator, and sent me off in search of a flat-bladed knife, she'd had Jamie Whitton in mind. And she was right. He kept his end up gamely all day long. "I never even touched it." "I guessed what was in it, anyway." "You two are just stupid." But after the last bell rang, Tulip hurried me across the playground and behind the wall.

"Keep your head down."

"Why?"

"Just *wait*!" she said fiercely.

Obediently, I waited. Cars pulled up outside the school. Doors slammed. Cars drove away.

"Now!" she said. "Take a look!"

She'd timed it perfectly. Just as we raised our heads, Jamie's mother slid the car into gear and pulled out from the kerb. And though, when he spotted us watching, he turned his head away as fast as possible, I still had time to see, through the freshly-washed windscreen, the first few fat tears of misery roll down his cheek.

And, when I turned to look at her, Tulip's smile.

And there's another time I shan't forget, when I cut my knee, wading over to the stone boy in the lily pond. I was carrying a hat we had spent hours dressing with feathers, so I didn't dare use my hands to save myself when I stumbled and fell against the sharp side of his pedestal.

Blood poured from the gash. I looked down and felt quite frightened. With each step I took against the water, blood washed away, then welled again.

"Hurry!" yelled Tulip. "Walk faster! Run!"

No one can run through water. By the time I got back to the edge, my heart was thumping. Tulip prised the hat from my hands. It wasn't even splashed.

"Good heavens, child!"

One of the guests had strolled over to see what was happening. Scattering peacocks, she hurried me up the terrace and propped me against a ledge. First came a linen cloth from one of the bars. I soaked that scarlet in seconds. Then came the towels. And then my parents arrived.

Tulip danced round, getting in everyone's way as Dad went to fetch a car as close as he could without flattening the flower beds, and everyone else spilled out advice.

"You realise she'll need at least half a dozen stitches."

"I shouldn't bother with the surgery. I'd take her straight to Casualty at the hospital."

"Don't worry, Mrs Barnes. These things so often look a whole lot worse than they are."

Dad appeared round the corner. Behind him, a car engine throbbed. I was handed down over the terrace, and Mum ran to keep up as Dad strode with me in his arms towards the back seat. He tipped me in, and Mum threw herself in beside me and slammed the door after her.

Someone opened the door again, to push in more towels.

"Oh, thank you!" said Mum. "Thank you!"

I heard a sharp tap, and looked through the other window. Tulip was just outside, prancing about like a monkey. She made a stupid face, splaying her hands, tipping her head sideways and sticking out her tongue.

Turning away, I caught the look my mother gave her in return. I shut my eyes then. I can shut them now. But I can still see both their faces.

Tulip's? Well, ugly and uncaring, certainly.

But Mum's?

Far, far more disturbing, somehow. I can't really explain. All I can tell you is that Mum was looking at Tulip the way no one normally looks at a child.

Twelve

BUT TULIP WAS always doing stupid things. Soon she was spending as much time sitting outside Miss Golightly's office as she spent back in class. And one day, chatting to Dad while he was doing the monthly cellar check, I very carelessly let this slip.

Dad casually changed the subject. But I knew what I'd said struck home. For two days, nothing happened. But then Will Stannard came back into class from the dentist to report that my dad's car was parked right outside the school.

Next morning, Mr Barraclough walked in and said, "I think we'll sit you next to Barney, Natalie."

Tulip was outraged.

"Why does she have to move?"

Mr Barraclough bit back a sharp response, and said instead:

"We all just think that everyone might benefit from a little change."

Furious, Tulip swept everything off her desk onto the floor.

"If Natalie can't sit by me, then I'm not doing any more work!"

If any of the rest of us had done that, we would have been in such deep trouble. But it was as if the staff were half-scared, half-despairing of Tulip. So Mr Barraclough let her be. She sat, stone-faced, arms folded, through the lesson, and he ignored her. When the bell rang, he sent her to the office as usual. And I spent yet another lonely break. None of the other children would come near me. Tulip's sheer reckless-ness made them nervous, too. And if there was even the slightest possibility that she might be sent back out in time to join us, they'd always take the precaution of staying clear.

In class time, to be fair, the teachers tried over and over to give me opportunities to make new friends.

"Natalie, why don't you pair up with Susan to put up the new corridor display?"

"Marcie and Natalie, I'll leave you here to set out all the chairs."

I'd chat to them, and they'd chat back. I'd even

wonder what it would be like to have them as friends. But when we came back in the classroom I couldn't help but glance across. And there was Tulip, seeking me out with her hard, hungry little eyes, as if she could actually *see* if I'd stayed faithful, if I still belonged to her. Back then, of course, I never thought to wonder what it was Tulip saw in me. But now I think, could some small part of it have been that, if she could keep someone as faceless and nondescript as me as her friend, then it really couldn't prove so much that everyone else hated her?

And hate her they did. Because she spoiled *everything*.

"I'm afraid we can't start until Tulip's quite ready."

"If there's any more messing about, then we won't have the ropes out – *Tulip!*"

"I'm sorry if it's a disappointment to most of you, but after a certain person's behaviour on the last field trip . . ."

The staff lost patience with her.

"Why do you make things so difficult for yourself?"

She'd scowl, but not answer, making that old game of ours, *Days of Dumbness*, into a regular thing.

"I'm still waiting . . ."

Still no response. People from other classes would walk past in the corridor and eye her curiously.

"You do realise, don't you, Tulip, that this is just one more silly way of trying to grab everyone's attention. But there are a lot of people in this school. Not just you."

Another few minutes of silence, and then whichever teacher it was would usually crack.

"Well, you'd better go out for break now. And when you come in again, I expect you to be more sensible. Off you go."

Out in the playground, she'd run wild, swearing and shrieking, and cheeking the dinner ladies, while I stood by, passively watching.

One day a message came, bellowed out from the steps, and picked up excitedly by everyone round me.

"Natalie! Miss Golightly wants you in her room. Right now!"

"Miss Golightly wants Natalie!"

"Natalie, you've got to go to the office."

"Not just to the office. Miss Golightly wants to see her!"

"Hurry, Natalie!"

The world drained of colour. I was terrified. I stumbled on the steps, and got lost round corners I knew as well as my own face. With the secretary watching, I tapped on the panels of Miss Golightly's door.

"Is that Natalie Barnes?"

Timidly, I pushed. But already Miss Golightly was striding towards me. Thrusting the door wide, she caught me by the neck of my jersey, and hauled me across to the window.

"Is that your friend?" she cried, pointing. "Is it? *Is* it?"

Tulip was running up to gangs of little ones, and stamping at their games.

"Look at her! Spoiling things for everybody! Rampaging about!"

She made a visible effort to calm herself.

"Sit down, Natalie. It's time that you and I had a little talk."

I don't remember much of it. Only how very frightened I was suddenly to be put in a chair that had cushions, and talked to as if I were grown up. It seemed to break all the rules, and left me too rattled even to listen properly, let alone speak up with sensible answers. Only when Miss Golightly moved on from

63

what she kept calling 'Tulip's real difficulties' and her 'influence on the people around her' did I stop feeling like a panicked rabbit. By then, she must have been hinting at my parents' concerns, because the first words I remember saying were:

"They can't mind Tulip that much, because they let her come."

She looked astonished.

"What? To the Palace? Really?"

"Yes," I said resolutely. "She comes a lot. Dad's very nice to her."

This irritated Miss Golightly, you could tell. Clearly Dad must have given her a very different picture.

Frowning, she said, "Perhaps they prefer to keep an eye on the two of you together. Have you thought of that?"

Dutifully, I tried to look as if she might be right. But I knew better. I'd worked out long ago that Mum let Tulip keep coming because she couldn't stand watching me mope round the Palace without her. It just got on her nerves to see me floating aimlessly through room after room. And Dad had a soft spot for Tulip. He knew her faults. And he may even have thought she was as bad for me outside school as she was in. But I'd seen the look on his face the day we drove round a corner to find Mr Pierce thrashing his dog in the shadow of a hedgerow. And I saw the extra gentleness and courtesy with which he always greeted Tulip's mother when she tried creeping past us in the street. Dad didn't say much. But I knew exactly what he thought of Tulip's home life.

And tell her she couldn't come? Well, he just couldn't do it.

Perhaps Miss Golightly thought he'd not been straight with her, with his complaints. In any case, my ticking off was over. She rose to her feet.

"Natalie, I hope you'll think seriously about all the things I've been saying." This time the hand on my shoulder was almost gentle as she walked me to the door. "Because, I warn you, you'll come to no good at all as Tulip's hold-your-coat merchant. Think about that."

Tulip was lying in wait in the playground.

"What did she want?"

My heart was back to thumping.

"Nothing much, honestly."

Tulip was irritated.

"Well, then, Birdbrain, what did she *say*?"

Perhaps I was peeved with her for getting me into

such trouble. Anyhow, just for once I managed to speak up for myself.

"I don't think that birdbrains are bright enough to remember what's been said to them."

Furious, she lashed out at the nearest thing, which was a folding sign about the next parents' evening. One of the dinner ladies bore down on her threateningly, and I vanished round the corner. I wandered nervously round the edges of the infants' playing area. But by the time Tulip ambled back in sight, accompanied by Marcie, she was all smiles. I wondered if she'd forgotten I'd been somewhere of interest, though I had more sense than to resurrect the subject. But that night, when Mum sent me along to give George the barman a message, I sidled up to one of the guests I knew best on my way out, and asked him,

"Mr Scott Henderson, what's a hold-your-coat merchant?"

Winking at George, he said to me, "Now don't you tell me that you and your little friend are getting into fights!"

I felt myself go scarlet.

"Fights?"

"That's what it means," he explained. "A hold-your-coat merchant is a person who likes to watch someone else get into trouble." He made his voice sound like a little boy's. "'Go on!'" he squeaked. "'You fight him! He deserves it! I'll stand here safely and I'll hold your coat.'"

He took a sip of whisky.

"Why are you asking, anyway?"

I'm not allowed to linger in the bars, and just as I began to scour my brain for some likely story, George raised his eyebrows at me over the beer glass he was polishing.

I danced away.

"No reason," I carolled behind me. "It just came up at school."

Next morning, I learned the reasons for Tulip's smiles. I kept my eyes peeled for her all the way from the nursery. But when I reached the school gates, she was already in the playground, locked arm in arm with Marcie.

She greeted me coolly.

"Marcie's with us today. That's all right, isn't it?"

I nodded. Marcie's quarrels with Claire, though frequent and explosive, were famously short-lived. I thought that I'd have Tulip back by break. But Marcie stayed with us all day. I was upset. (Tulip kept calling me Birdbrain.) But still I tagged along, pretending I hardly noticed and didn't care, till we drifted past Harry's supermarket after school.

"Coming in?"

You could tell from her eyes it was a challenge.

"No," I said. "Not today."

"Why not?"

"He watches us. I can feel it. He doesn't like us in there."

"That's *his* problem."

"But it makes me not want to go in there."

"Baby!"

But Marcie was tugging on her arm, so she gave up and we went round the back. We started balancing along the low walls dividing the sections of the car park. Right in the middle of a wobbly arabesque, Tulip suddenly announced to Marcie that the manager of Harry's had that very morning offered her a Saturday job.

"Don't be silly," said Marcie. "Nobody gives that sort of work to somebody our age."

"It's supposed to be unofficial. He said I remind him of his little sister, who choked to death on pencil sharpenings."

On pencil sharpenings! The Tulip touch! I was so mad at her for the sheer stupidness of it (and for ignoring me so horribly) that when she took a gold chain I'd never seen before out of her pocket and twirled it round her fingers, I left it to Marcie to ask all the questions.

"Where did you get that?"

"It's mine."

"Is it gold, though? Real gold?"

"Of course it is."

"Can I see it?"

"You're looking at it."

"No, I mean, can I hold it?"

Pleased with her interest, Tulip spilled the chain into Marcie's hand. Marcie turned to the sunlight and studied it.

"This *is* real gold. It's got that funny mark." She raised her eyes to Tulip's. "It can't be yours."

"Yes, it is."

"I don't think so. It must be worth an awful lot."

The edgy tone I knew so well came into Tulip's voice.

"Why shouldn't it be mine?"

Marcie said nothing, and, with Tulip standing there

69

in her cheap clothes and worn jacket, there was no need.

Furious, Tulip snatched back the necklace and hurled it, glinting and rippling, as far as she could. It flew across the car park like a live snake, and fell with a rattle into the huge rubbish drum beside the wall.

We stared. Then Tulip said to Marcie,

"I don't want it any more. You can have it if you find it."

Marcie hesitated just a shade too long. And then, humiliated by the notion of scrabbling in a dustbin for something cast out by Tulip, she turned her back on us.

"I don't want it!"

She strode away without another word. Part of me so longed to follow. I knew that I could catch her by the arm, and say to her, "I reckon Tulip must have *stolen* that," and in the sheer excitement of the moment, we could have become friends. I even thought that when she made up again with Claire, she very probably would let me stay.

I was still staring after her forlornly when Tulip said,

"I'm going home now."

I walked with her as far as the bridge. We still

weren't friendly. In fact, we hardly spoke. All I remember is that, at one point, she was struggling to find something at the bottom of her schoolbag, and things kept dropping, so she turned to me.

"Here," she said. "Be some help, will you? Hold my coat."

PART
Two

One

I T WAS JULIUS who started it. We were sitting on the wall of the verandah one morning, poring over his spelling book, when he said suddenly,

"Did you know Tulip was a witch?"

"Don't be silly."

"She is," he said stubbornly. "She always knows exactly what I'm thinking."

"No one knows what you're thinking."

"Tulip does."

"Can we get on with these, please? *Wheelbarrow*."

He reeled it off, "W..h..e..e..l..b..a..r..r..o..w," and went on without a break. "She knew which cake I wanted yesterday. When Mum sent the plate round, Tulip was reading my mind to see which one I was after. Then she took it."

"I expect you were staring at it."

"No," he said gravely. "I used to be that silly. But

I stopped doing that ages ago, and made it so I only *thought*." He shifted uncomfortably on the ledge. "Then she got good at that as well."

"Good at what?"

"Knowing what I was thinking."

"Julius –"

"And then," he finished in a rush, "I learned to make myself think something different. If I want the only coconut cake on the plate, I think 'I want the chocolate one' as hard as I can. And, for a while, it fooled her."

He laced his fingers, and bent them back nervously.

"But not any more. She can get through that too, now. She can read what I really think."

And there was no shaking him. Tulip was a witch. And that's what must have set me off. From that day on, I lost my confidence that all the thoughts I had were quite my own. At first, it started as a little game. (Not one of the ones we did together. A private one I never shared with her.) I'd make believe that, if she wanted, she could read my mind, and even send her own thoughts directly into my head, to swirl about and make the whole place hers. I'd try and lay myself open to it, and be a blank slate in case it really could happen. And that felt so weird and puppet-like that I came to enjoy it. Soon, even when we were busy with other things, I'd secretly be playing *The Tulip Touch*, practically inviting her in.

"Want to play *All the Grey People*?" she'd ask me.

"Whatever you want."

"I'll be the leader, shall I?"

"Yes. You be leader."

"Right. First, we'll go through the coffee lounge. And then the writing room. And then the conservatory."

"All right."

You'd think I didn't have a will of my own. And wouldn't you suspect that she'd get bored, playing with such a servile shadow? But not a bit of it. It suited her fine. We'd march in silence through the chosen rooms, gazing with utter contempt at all those amazingly dull-looking people who spent an age tinkling their coffee cups, or staring into space over their drinks, or fiddling inside their handbags. Did they have any thoughts at all? Could they be thinking interesting things? Or were they just as they seemed – people with brains as grey and lifeless as their faces?

Dad spotted us on our third circuit.

"Okay, you two. Hop along. These rooms are supposed to be restful."

And off we went, to play *Along the Flaggy Shore* in the upstairs passage, or *Fat and Loud* outside the bar. Whatever Tulip felt like doing next. She must have noticed I was different. But she never said a word. Even back then, that bothered me. What did she *think* was happening? And once I remember turning back, when she had sent me off across the hall to snaffle a few sheets of headed paper from the desk. And she had such a horrid smile on her face. Smug, she looked. Cocky.

I fetched the paper. But when I came back, my self-imposed reflex of submission failed.

"I don't see why *I* had to get it."

"Oh, don't you?"

The tone was disdainful. And the look said, clear as paint: 'I know why you chose *me*. But surely, surely, even someone as stupid as you has worked out by now why it was someone like me chose *you*.'

TWO

EXPLAIN TO ME how you can come so close to rescue, only to have it snatched away. Just take the time when we were moving up together from the village school to Talbot Harries, in town. I didn't realise anything was brewing till Dad made a point of seeking me and Tulip out.

"So what are you two young ladies up to today?"

Tulip stood up and brushed the grass bits from her knees. We'd been in the middle of *Guest-stalk* (not one of the games we admitted to playing), and he'd blown our cover by walking straight up to us. Our prey strolled off.

"Nothing much. Why?"

"No reason."

He gazed round, casually. It was quite obvious that he was after something, but not sure if he had the time to work it in the conversation gradually. Then one of the waiters appeared on the verandah to give him a quick 'You're needed in the restaurant' signal.

Dad came directly to the point.

"Which school are you moving on to after the holidays, Tulip? Is it Talbot Harries?"

She made a face.

"I suppose so. No one's said anything different."

Now the waiter was back again. It was quite obvious there was a difficult guest inside.

"You'll still be with Natalie, then," Dad told her cheerfully. And then, "Excuse me, girls," as he hurried back across the lawn. I couldn't look at Tulip. Suddenly, like someone drowning, I wanted so much to lift an arm to try and save myself. And Tulip could always read my face. If I knew Dad was lying, she'd know it too.

"Look at the peacocks," I said. "I hate the stupid way they walk."

Tulip ignored me.

"If he's planning on separating us," she said thoughtfully, "he'll have to put more effort into it than that."

That night, I overheard the plan.

"I think we should send Natalie to Heathcote."

"To Heathcote? But *why*?"

"Why not? I know it's a lot further, but several children from the village go there."

He saw me watching them and lowered his voice. Taking Mum's arm, he led her into the office. I didn't hear the rest. But over the next few days, Mum tried again and again to sound me out.

"How would you feel about it, Natalie? It's a long bus ride."

I shrugged.

"You'd see a lot less of –" She hesitated. "Some of your old friends."

I shrugged again. I knew if I was sent to Heathcote, that would be curtains for mornings and evenings with Tulip. I'd set off too early and get back too late. It wasn't clear why it should make a difference to week-ends. (It wasn't, after all, as if Tulip had hordes of admirers aching to step in and take my place.) But surely in a new school, with new teachers, new class-mates, new people on the bus, I would be able to make new friends.

The registration forms sat in the in-tray on the reception desk. I fingered them over and over when no one was watching. *Heathcote Grange Secondary School. Last date for applications: Thursday 18th August.*

I could have filled it in myself, it was so easy. *Name. Home address(es). Date of birth. Previous schools. Names and ages of siblings. Health problems (if any).*

The days before the deadline, I was a bird on a hot wire. Each time Dad came through a doorway, or cleared his throat, I was expecting him to say,

"Well, it's decided, Natalie. Heathcote, it is."

On Monday, the wrong meat orders were delivered, and two of the waiters fell out and stormed off work. On Tuesday, Julius got a lump of grit in his eye, and rubbed it so hard he had to be taken down to the surgery. Wednesday was kitchen inspection. Everything stops for that. And on Thursday, though I hung around, wondering if Dad would suddenly come bounding down the steps ("You might as well see the place, Natalie. Why don't you come along for the ride?"), nothing happened. No one went anywhere. And when I fingered through the papers in the tray, I saw the form was still quite blank.

Tulip turned up next morning for the first time in a week. Dad met her on the stairs and suddenly looked troubled. She gave him her usual cheeky grin.

"Morning, Mr Barnes."

"Hello, Tulip."

Lightly, she bounced her fingers on the banisters,

and carried on up. He hurried down. I watched him make for the reception desk and riffle through the in-tray.

Mum came out of the office.

"What's that you're looking for?"

He held it up.

"Oh, dear," she said. "Oh, what a nuisance! What's the date on it?"

"The eighteenth. Yesterday."

"No point in driving it in, and begging them to take her anyway?"

He looked at his watch.

"The Newsams will be here in ten minutes to sort out the details of their wedding lunch."

"I could do that with them."

"I thought you were taking Julius for his check-up."

"Oh. Right."

There was a worried pause. I watched from overhead. Tulip was watching me. And suddenly I knew beyond a shadow of a doubt that she had stayed away all week deliberately, to lower their guard.

Mum shook off her unease.

"It's not too late, I'm sure. Shall we think about it as soon as we've got a free moment?"

Dad noticed Tulip lingering on the stairs.

"Yes. Later," he said, and hurried off. And that was the last I heard. The form lay in the tray another week, and then it vanished. The last days disappeared as well. (We found a skylight with a smashed alarm, and played *Watch the Skies* behind the parapets.) And on the first day of September I turned up at the bus stop. New journey. New uniform. New school. New set of teachers.

And good old Tulip, as usual.

Three

I HATED TALBOT Harries. So did she. Hated the slime-green rooms, the shoving corridors, the ringing cloakrooms and the screaming bells. Hated the work, and hated the sarcastic teachers. Hated the food.

And hated being on my own. Someone had shopped us. We never found out if it was Dad, or the teachers from our old school. But we were separated for almost every lesson. Even our registration class was not the same. I'd catch a glimpse of Tulip as she was buffeted my way down some seething staircase, and call out hopefully,

"See you at break on the back steps!"

But she was hardly ever there, and each school hour went on for ever, till I was a bag of nerves who jumped at every raised voice in a corridor, and bit my fingernails until they bled, and couldn't concentrate on what the teachers said for the hot tears prickling behind my eyes.

"This is your fault!" I shouted at Julius, when he caught me weeping over homework I couldn't do. "If it weren't for you and your stupid sore eye, I'd be at Heathcote now!"

He backed away. I wondered if he'd gone to tell on me. But, no. He came back a few minutes later with a heap of mint imperials he'd pinched from the bowl in the coffee lounge. While I sucked for comfort, Julius patted me. And though it made it harder than ever to concentrate on the homework, I couldn't bring myself to shake him off. It wasn't Julius's fault that he was the apple of Mum's eye, and everything to do with him came first and second and next and last. Julius's tumbling class. Julius's visit to the clinic. New trousers for Julius. He didn't set it off, or even encourage it. Mum had no need of that. It hadn't escaped anybody's attention that even though furry rabbit and poor, battered Mr Haroun had long ago been tossed up on the shelf of precious cast-off cuddly things, Mum never did grow out of Julius. Even when he was dying to scramble out of the car, his fingers rattling the handle and his face turned to go, she'd be hungrily reaching out for him.

"Say goodbye properly, darling. Give Mummy one last hug."

At least he never smirked or crowed at always coming first. Sometimes he even looked rueful, as if I'd been the luckier of the two, with no one noticing if I was there or not, or if I was happy, or if things were going right or wrong.

"Sorry," I sniffled again. And he turned up the patting.

"I know," he said. "I'll go and tell them you're crying."

It was a generous offer. It's never easy in a big hotel to get attention (if you're not paying for it). But if it was Julius who went, Mum would look up at once.

I shook my head.

"No. Honestly. I'll be all right."

And no doubt I soon was. It's hard for anyone to start at a new school. Tiring and nerve-wracking. No wonder I was always so glad to see Tulip waiting on the steps at ten to four.

I'd rush up, full of questions.

"Where *were* you? You can't have been in your gym class. I went past twice, and didn't see you through the glass. Were you hiding in the cloakroom?"

She'd give her little sideways grin.

"Tell you later. Let's just get out of here."

She'd take my arm, and off we'd go past all the people who'd come on with us from our old school. Susan and Janet, with their brand new friends, and Will and Jamie, who'd been accepted at once in the 'Lads' Gang'. We'd saunter down the street towards our stop.

I'd hear a rumble gathering behind us.

"Here's a bus coming now."

She'd cock her head to one side.

"What's it to be, then? Home or *Havoc*?"

And so relieved to be out of there, out at last, and no longer alone, I'd choose the one I knew she wanted to hear.

"*Havoc!*" I'd cry. "*Havoc!*"

And as the bus roared past, with the breeze of it whipping up our skirts, we'd slip away down the alley, out of sight.

Four

YOU COULDN'T REALLY call it havoc. It was just stupid things like cheeking people as we ran past, and telling old ladies their short cut was closed at the other end because the police had found a body with its throat cut, and hiding behind walls to flick mud pellets at women wearing smart jackets. ("Don't waste any of them on the men," Tulip ordered. "Men never bother, anyway.")

Sometimes we were spiteful. When the young mothers poured out of the playgroup centre into the post office shop, we'd stand in front of the display of foreign stamps till everyone's back was turned. Then Tulip would jam one of her specially selected twigs – short, but tough and sinewy – between the spokes of the nearest parked pushchair. Casually, we'd move into the queue, and watch with glee as the frustrated mother pushed and tugged, and struggled with the brake. Once, we watched one of them burst into tears, and I felt bad. But mostly I took Tulip's line on it. It was just 'fun', 'a good laugh', 'something to do'.

I only stopped her twice. Once, when she started with the milk bottle smashing. And another time, when she took someone's rabbit out of its hutch.

We'd had fun with animals before. Dead ones. It's not till you go looking that you have any idea how many dead birds and furry things are lying round the average town. (Sometimes I think I'll never be able to see another road kill without thinking of Tulip.) She'd flick them over with her shoe.

"Looks all right to me," she'd say critically. "Yes. That'll do."

She'd scoop it up in one of the torn plastic bags with which Urlingham is littered, and we'd carry it round with us – it could have been a loaf and a pound of tomatoes – until we saw the perfect place.

"There's a hutch."

We'd be up to the fence in a moment.

"Is it empty?"

"Doesn't matter."

It wouldn't have, either. I'd watched her push fat, spoiled rabbits off their favourite patch of straw to shove a dead pigeon or blackbird in their place. But,

"I meant the *house*," I said.

"Oh, that." She glanced dismissively at the kitchen window with its prissy curtains hanging in scallops. "There's no one looking, anyway."

I checked the upstairs windows. But there were no signs of life, no shadows moving back and forth.

"Who's going, then?"

"I'll go."

I gave her a leg up. There was no stopping Tulip once she'd started, so it was better to get the whole business done. She landed lightly on the other side. I passed the mucky bag over, and she set off boldly, sauntering across the lawn as if she owned it.

I watched her prise open the hutch lid.

"Well, hello, Thumper."

She lifted the rabbit out by the ears. I hated that. I knew people said it didn't hurt them, but I didn't believe it. And there was something in the way she did it – slowly, deliberately, almost with relish – that set my nerves on edge, and started me scrambling along the fence, looking for a foothold of my own.

By the time I got over, she had her hands over its eyes.

"Gone dark, has it, Bunny?"

You had to be careful. She could turn just like that. So:

"Can I hold him, Tulip? Just for a little bit?"

She shook her head.

"First come, first served."

"Please," I said. "Give him to me."

She grinned unpleasantly.

"You don't know he's a he. He might be a she."

"It doesn't matter. You could just let me have a go at cuddling him."

"Only if you've guessed right."

She upturned the squirming rabbit for no more than a couple of seconds.

"She's a she. So she's mine."

"She's not *yours*, Tulip."

"She is now."

Tulip was crooning in the rabbit's ear. "Who's a clever bunny? Who's going to be a good girl? Who's Tulip's special one? She's not going to make a fuss, is she? Oh, no. She isn't going to do that. Because she enjoys it really, doesn't she? And if she starts struggling, she'll get *hurt*."

She finished up so savagely that I knew I was watching something horrible, nothing to do with the rabbit she was holding, but darker, much darker, and hidden, and coming from deep inside Tulip.

I heard my own voice saying,

"Put it *down*!"

It was like breaking a spell. The strange look cleared from her face. She practically threw the rabbit back on its straw, and turned away. I slammed the hutch lid closed.

"Quick!" I said. "Someone's watching! Hurry up!"

She wasn't fooled. To prove it, she very deliberately took her time, snapping heads off the flowers as she strolled back towards the fence. I didn't care. I just scrambled over as fast as I could, and then, fuelled with relief at landing on the other side, gave myself over to her yet again.

"What shall we do now, Tulip? You decide."

Five

THAT WAS THE year we started *The Little Visits*. I've no idea what set us off. All I remember is that one minute we were rollicking merrily, arm in arm, past some perfect stranger's front gate. And the next, we were on the doorstep, and Tulip had her finger pressed firmly on the ringing bell.

"Yes? Can I help you?"

I'm no good at ages. She was older than Mum, and younger than most people's grannies.

"We were wondering if you could tell us the way to the castle."

"Castle?" The woman looked baffled. "There's no castle round here."

"Url Castle," persisted Tulip.

It sounded so silly, I nearly let out a snigger.

"No. Not round here."

But neither of us moved. And, in the end, she let us in the hall. While she leafed through a stack of pamphlets from a drawer, we rolled our eyes and made sneering faces at one another about the pictures on her walls.

"I'm sorry," she said at last, looking up. "I can find nothing here."

But Tulip didn't move, so neither did I.

"You'll have to go now, I'm afraid," the woman said after a moment.

I watched Tulip meet her gaze and willed her not to push her luck and get us into trouble. But then Tulip put on her false smile.

"Thank you for looking, anyway."

Hastily, I slapped on my dad's be-pleasant-to-the-guests face.

"Yes. Thank you for looking."

She was still staring when we turned at the gate.

"Goodbye," Tulip called out sweetly. "Thank you again."

The woman didn't move. I wondered if somehow, by accident, Tulip had picked a particularly suspicious person, or if, at the next house she chose, there'd be somebody even more wary and watchful.

"Your turn," said Tulip. She made me run up and

down the street till my face was sticky and burning. Then I knocked on the door.

"Excuse me for bothering you. But could I please come in and have a glass of water?"

The elderly gentleman ran his eyes over my school uniform, as if to assure himself it wasn't fake.

"You needn't come in. I'll fetch some water. Just stay there."

There was an edge to his voice, and he glanced round twice as he hurried to the kitchen. I knew if I so much as stepped over the wooden strip dividing indoors from out, he'd shoot back, whether or not the glass was filled, and order me away.

The tumbler he handed me was clouded and knobbly.

"There you are."

He stood and waited. I took a couple of sips. Tulip had assured me that, if I could only get the person chatting, I'd be inside in a flash. So I said,

"We have some glasses just like this at home."

"Do you?" he said coldly.

We don't, of course. The glasses at the Palace are crystal clear. Always shining. Always sparkling.

"Please hurry and drink it. I have things to do."

I saw Tulip watching me from over the hedge.

"It's hard to drink fast," I said hastily. "The problem's with my throat. With swallowing. Last time I was in hospital, they thought they'd got rid of it. It's very unusual, you see, in someone my age. So everyone was very disappointed when it came back."

And I was in, of course. I only stayed a few minutes, till I felt 'a little less dizzy'.

But I'd got in.

Six

GRADUALLY, OVER THE months, Tulip set harder and harder tasks.

"May I please use your telephone?"

"Do you have a biscuit for my friend?"

"Would you lend me a pencil and some paper?"

It was astonishing, sometimes, just how easy it was. Some people didn't even count, said Tulip. They were obviously so lonely that if we'd been wearing masks and carrying knives, they'd still probably have ushered us into their kitchens. Others were bewildered or suspicious, which made it that bit harder to tack on the extras Tulip insisted on, like taking advantage of the house owner's back being turned to swivel a framed photo round to face the wall, or slide their scissors off the table and stab them, points down, in the soil of a plant pot.

We never stayed too long, though. Just in case.

And, even so, I sometimes got home late. Usually, no one noticed. (It's not as if I walk through the main door and ask for my key at Reception.) But sometimes, slipping silently up the back stairs, I'd bump into Mum and see her glance curiously at her watch.

"Miss the bus, darling?"

"It was silly," I'd say. "Marcie and I got chatting, and then Mr Phillips wanted something carrying round to the laboratories, and . . ."

My voice trailed off, even before the next set of doors could swallow it entirely. She never called me back to hear the end. I doubt if she was listening, anyway. Always, in a hotel, there are dozens of things to get done. She was forever busy. And often I was glad of that. After Tulip invented *Wild Nights*, it might be hours before my heart stopped thudding, and I stopped being certain, each time the phone rang, that it was the fire service or the police.

I don't know why *Wild Nights* came as such a surprise. Tulip had always had a passion for fire. Candles, matches, sparklers, bonfires – she loved them all. I can't count the number of times Dad caught her behind the dustbins setting fire to paper just to watch it blaze, then flush with orange sprinkles as it crumpled to black at her feet. Give her some fancy wrapping paper, and she'd sit for hours tearing it into strips, and dropping them, one by one, into the fire in the back lounge.

"Look! Look at this greeny-blue!"

"Just like the peacocks' fans."

Her face glowed with scorn in the firelight.

"No, no. It's much greener and bluer than that. These colours are *magic*."

We helped with every bonfire. Well, I helped. She simply poked holes through the sodden leaves, and watched the red caves deep inside them burn.

"Come on, Tulip. I've fetched three whole bags while you've been standing there."

"Ssh! Don't bother me."

The gardener used to nudge me. "Don't go too close," he'd say. "Can't you see Tulip's worshipping her fire god?"

It was a joke. But, honestly, you might have thought she was in church, the way she stayed so still, grave-faced and silent. Not like on *Wild Nights*. When we played that, some sort of unholy excitement ran through her every gesture, her every word. She'd push and pull me to the place she had in mind, while I begged not to go.

"Oh, please, Tulip. Let's just catch the bus straight home."

"You're a coward and a lily-liver!" And sometimes worse. Once, a man passing by heard her swearing at me so foully, he stopped to stare.

She made a face at him, and pushed me on.

"We'll get in trouble," I wailed.

"So?"

And I was quiet, because, for me, the notion of getting in trouble was so serious that I had to hide from her exactly how much it mattered. And she wouldn't have understood, anyhow. Things were so different at her house. Tulip said very little, but I'd picked up the fact that she was always being punished for stupid things like knocking a fork off the table, or leaving a stiff tap dripping a tiny bit, or not coming quickly enough when Mr Pierce called her. Her dad would suddenly let fly, and keep at her till even her timid mother was forced to stop pretending she hadn't noticed what was going on. She'd step in to try and stop him. Then Mr Pierce would turn his savage mood on her.

"It makes no difference what I do," Tulip explained. "He picks on me to start a fight with her."

So there was no stopping her by wailing about 'trouble'. She simply grabbed handfuls of my coat, and pulled again.

"Come on, Natalie! It's all planned."

Sometimes I'd trawl around for an excuse.

"No, not tonight. I promised Mum I'd help with next week's menus."

Tipping her head to the side, she'd say sarcastically:

"Does the itsy-bitsy baby want to go home to her mummy?"

I hated it when she jeered at me.

"All right," I said. "But only something small."

"A Sweetie Swipe?"

"No. He watches us every minute, Tulip. He *knows*."

"All right, then. Exploding Greenhouse."

"No!"

She made her last offer. "Dustbin fire! It's only rubbish, anyway."

"All right. A dustbin fire. But only *one*."

"Only one."

"Promise, Tulip."

"Cross my heart."

Her eyes went wide with honest promising, just as, in half an hour's time, they'd widen again from all the spitting orange magic conjured from some perfect stranger's matching grey bins.

"Tulip, you promised! *One*, you said."

"I meant one *more*, Stupid!"

She was so horrid to me. Endlessly rude and disparaging. But, somehow, it didn't hurt. I think I just treated her insults like bad weather, keeping my head down, and pressing on with my self-appointed task of keeping her out of trouble. It was I who prised the package she was about to send to Mrs Bodell out of her hand.

"You can't post that!"

"Why not?"

"You're not allowed to put stuff like that in a letter box."

I hurled it as far as it would go into the road, and watched with satisfaction as a car rolled over it.

"Good job I didn't bother with a stamp," she said, unruffled.

In the same way, I confiscated her rude Christmas cards, one by one, as she finished them.

"Tulip, it's such a *waste*. You spend ages doing all this brilliant lettering, and I have to rip them into pieces and stuff them in the bin."

"Nobody makes you."

And it was true. Nobody made me. But still, somehow, I'd come to believe that keeping Tulip out of the trouble she spent her whole life fomenting was time well spent. And maybe it was, for me. It kept me close to her, and I needed Tulip. While I trailed round quietly, doing what I was told and being no trouble, Tulip lived my secret life. While teachers watched me sitting quietly at my desk, I was really outside on the hill with Tulip, openly watching the rest of us file in and out of classes. When I answered the Palace guests' boring questions over and over again, always polite, always smiling, I was secretly swearing as foully as she did. And when Mum didn't notice me as she swept past, looking for Julius, I was in silent rages that would put Tulip to shame.

I was as bad as she was, and the clever thing was, nobody even noticed. Even Dad was fooled.

"You're looking pale. Are you sure that you're sleeping properly?"

"I'm all right."

He turned me round to the light.

"But you've got shadows underneath your eyes."

"I've been doing a lot of homework."

"Tell me another!" he scoffed. But you could tell that he believed me. And why not? It was a whole lot easier, and took less time, than trying to find out the truth.

Seven

SPRING CAME, AND Tulip's moods got worse and worse. She swung doors in my face, and kicked a huge dent in my cloakroom locker, and was so hateful that even I took to steering clear of her for days on end. Then I'd walk in the girls' lavatories to find her scratching foul words on the wall over the sinks. And just as if we'd never been apart, I'd be back to trying to stop her.

"Tulip, they've only just finished painting in here. What's the point of making it look horrible straight away?"

She gouged the plaster with her locker key.

"It's their own fault! They shouldn't have chosen such a vile colour!"

"What's wrong with it?"

"It's stupid, that's what. Pink! Pink for nice little girlies!"

"It's better than that old green."

"I liked that green."

"You said you didn't. You were always going on about it."

Plaster sprayed from the wall.

"Oh, shut up, Natalie!"

She'd never had any patience, but now it seemed everything got under her skin. She was angry with everyone. And it didn't make any difference whether or not they were cross with her first. Almost as soon as anyone spoke to her, on went that little mask of frozen rage.

And when she wasn't angry, she was spiteful.

"That's rubbish, what you're drawing, Natalie."

I kept my eyes on my paper. Apart from Games, when we were often ordered into separate teams, Art was the only lesson we had together now.

"At least I don't draw the same thing every week."

And it was true. Give Tulip a piece of paper, and all she'd ever draw were children with huge, forlorn eyes copied from soppy greetings cards she'd lifted from the shop beyond the bus stop.

She moved her hand across to hide some now, because Mrs Minniver was coming our way.

"Have you started yet, Tulip?"

"I was just thinking first."

Mrs Minniver inspected her watch.

"You've got exactly half an hour. By the time that bell rings, I want to see a proper painting. None of your usual little self-pitying cherubs up in one corner. Every inch of that paper must be covered. Now get on with it."

Tulip turned to me sourly.

"So what is it?"

"What?"

"What we're supposed to be doing!"

"Self-portrait," I said coldly.

"Really?"

It seemed quite genuinely to be news to her. And, peaceably enough, she lifted her brush and pulled my tray of paints nearer her easel than mine, to start with her careless brush stabbings and pokings.

"Aren't you going to draw yourself first?"

"I know what I look like."

"But you'll go over the edges."

"I'm not doing it with edges."

I leaned across to see. She tugged her easel round, away from me. I went back to my own work. We sulked in silence for a little while. Well, *I* sulked. I think she just became absorbed in her painting. That horrid humming that she shared with her mother got on my nerves, but I didn't argue about it. I just kept hard at work, fretting about the face in my painting – too long, then too short, then too rubbed out and messy – till Kirstin strolled over to borrow a rubber and complain.

"That stupid Jeremy she's put me with! He's lost two of my rubbers already!"

"Well, look what I've got," Tulip said contemptuously.

I looked up. She was pointing at me.

And did I rise up and hit her? Did I slap her face? Send her wobbly easel flying and pour the scummy brush water over her head?

No. I just said feebly, "Oh, do shut up, Tulip!" and kept on with my work.

But I did hate her, then. I hated her so much that I could hardly wait for the half hour to disappear. I'd seen her fierce rubbings and scrubbings, her brutal daubs. Most people would take more care hurling rubbish into their dustbins. I'd seen her splayed brush come back again and again to the black, and what was left of the purple, and to the fiery red she'd turned to ditchwater with her careless rinsing. Suddenly I couldn't wait to see what Mrs Minniver made of Tulip's self-portrait.

The bell rang. She appeared in front of us.

"Finished?"

Tulip shrugged, totally indifferent, and tore her sheet of paper from the easel. Mrs Minniver took it from her. But though her face darkened as she inspected the painting, something about it must have given her pause, because she pinned it back on the easel and stepped back to look at it from further away.

And I stopped pretending that I wasn't watching, and looked at it too. It was the strangest thing. The fury and contempt of Tulip's brushwork had turned to whirlpools of violence on the paper. Everything about it was dark and furious, and every inch of it seemed to suck you in and swirl you round, making you feel dizzy and anxious. And everywhere you looked, your eyes were drawn back, over and over, to the centre, where, out of the blackness, two huge forlorn eyes stared out as usual, half-begging, half-accusing.

I waited for the explosion. Would it be 'wasting paper' or 'dumb insolence'? Or, 'I *warned* you, Tulip. No more self-pitying little staring round eyes'?

But Mrs Minniver just said,

"*Look* at it. Now that you've finished, at least take a *look*."

Putting her hands on Tulip's shoulders, she turned her to face the easel. Tulip's eyes went cold and hard. Mrs Minniver waited. But when it became obvious that Tulip wasn't going to say a word, she simply sighed.

"Well, then. Off you go," she said gently.

Tulip reached out to rip the painting off the easel, but Mrs Minniver put out a hand.

"No. I'll keep this."

Tulip stalked off. I stayed behind to pack her things along with mine, and ask,

"Will she get into trouble?"

Still staring distractedly at the painting, Mrs Minniver repeated,

"Trouble?"

"For making that huge mess," I insisted. "And doing more big round sad eyes, even though you told her that was exactly what she mustn't do."

I don't know what I expected. But certainly not a look of such contempt.

I felt so frustrated and betrayed. I could practically feel myself screaming inside. *Why does Tulip always get away with it? Why does nobody ever stop her? Why? Why? Why?*

But the best I could manage to Mrs Minniver was a sullen:

"It was supposed to be a self-portrait. That's what you *said*. A self-portrait. Nothing else!"

I waited for her to tell me off. 'Disloyalty to a friend'. 'Making trouble'. But she just turned back to the painting.

"Oh, Natalie," she said, as gently as she'd spoken to Tulip. "Look at it. Just *look* at it."

And this time it was there for me. My anger and frustration blew away like so much litter. I stood beside Mrs Minniver, staring at Tulip's self-portrait, and this time all that I could think was what I finally managed to whisper.

"Oh, Mrs Minniver! I'm just so glad that I'm not her."

Eight

So was it pity drew me back? Time and again, I'd almost gather up the strength to break away, and something would happen to stop me in my tracks. Like the day we heard the news about Muriel Brackenbury.

"Just think! We know somebody whose sister has drowned!"

"Tulip, stop *saying* that."

"But we could sell our stories to the paper. We could be photographed with our arms around Janet."

"Don't be ridiculous. Janet doesn't even like us."

Tulip's eyes shone.

"I bet she's so upset. She won't be able to stop thinking about it."

I was disgusted with her. Why was she so nosy about other people's feelings? Did she have none of her own, that she should be so obsessed about someone else's? And she didn't even feel sorry for Janet, that was obvious. She had the same look on her face as when we gave that horrible box to Jamie, and when she made Marcie cry by lying to her that she'd failed her maths. She just liked to prod and invent, and twist and poke, to watch people go ugly with fright, or burst into tears of misery.

Now she was rolling Muriel's name round and round.

"Brackenbury. Brackenbury. It's odd, isn't it? Because, I expect, when she was found, she was near bracken. And near berries."

"If you don't stop talking about it, I'm catching the next bus home."

She didn't even hear me.

"Drowned! Think of it. To get so close to the bank, and still go under. Swallowing all that water. I expect Janet will keep waking up imagining it now. I bet she will. After all, it's her sister."

"Don't Tulip! It's *horrible*."

"Yes, isn't it?"

I stared at her. She thought I meant 'horrible to drown', not 'horrible to say'. And settling herself on the wall by the bus stop, she just went on and on.

"It must feel awful, opening your mouth for air, and more and more water rushing in instead. I expect you swallow so much that, when they find you, you're all swollen up. Not like with kittens. I bet a person must keep trying, over and over, to –"

But I'd stopped listening. Everything round us – the street, the cars, the people – all bleached away to invisible. And I was back to eight years old, holding my father's hand on a baking afternoon, and seeing Tulip for the very first time, still as a stone in that cornfield.

Not yet a friend of hers. Not yet sucked in. And not in the slightest scared of her.

"You drowned that kitten, didn't you?"

She broke off her excited ramblings.

"Which kitten?"

"The one you were holding on the day we met. I always thought it was your dad who got rid of them. But it was you."

"No, it wasn't."

She said it quite firmly, though it wasn't true. But I was used to that. And suddenly I understood how Tulip could lie and lie, and never see how ridiculous her untruths looked to other people. In her eyes, it was the *world* that was wrong. If the world had only been right, if things had only fallen out the way they should, then she would never have had to lie, or steal, or be spiteful. If the world had only been right, she'd be a nice and good person – the girl she was inside, before it all went wrong, and she got spoiled all along with it.

"It *was* you," I persisted.

"So what if it was?"

"Nothing." I kept my voice easy, even bright. "I was just wondering, that's all."

"Wondering what?"

"What it was like."

She turned to look at me. I forced myself not to show even a flicker of feeling. I closed my mind to her. Slam! Clang! Shutters down! I wasn't going to play *The Tulip Touch* right now.

"It's none of your business."

"I know," I said. "It's just that I never realised. And you never said."

She gave the flippant playground retort.

"You never asked."

I felt like screaming at her, "Why should I ask, Tulip? Whoever would have even thought?" But, instead, I walked my fingers steadily along the wall, and tore off a strip of moss.

"Did it take long?" I asked, casually pulling the shreds apart.

Can you sense truth coming? Oh, I think you can.

"That's why I always had to do it myself," she said, firm, proud, self-righteous, even. "So it would take less time. They had to be done, you see, or we'd be *overrun*." I knew it was her father's word from the way that she said it. "*Overrun*. But Dad wouldn't take the time. He'd just shove them in a crock of water and slam the lid, and you could hear them scrabbling and pushing at the top. And it took forever."

I bet it did. I could hear it as I sat listening. The mewings and scratchings. The lid lifting like potatoes on the boil. The driblets of water down the side of the crock that only let in more air to prolong the struggle.

All her cocky self-confidence had drained away. She said so sadly:

"It took hours and hours."

I passed her half my moss. It sat on her skirt in a crumbling lump, but she didn't push it off.

"I did try to stop him. Once I even went at him with a fork. But he just laughed, and called me 'another little cat who could do with a ducking'. He didn't even bother to wallop me." (Even after all this

117

time, she sounded a little surprised.) "He just threw me out of the house, and rammed home the bolt. Then he sat with his feet on the table, reading the paper, and I had to watch through the window. It took hours and hours."

Her spongy bitten fingertips scrabbled for comfort in the moss.

"Not *hours*," I consoled her. "Kittens wouldn't be strong enough. Honestly. Not hours."

"Long enough," she said. "So ever since then I've always done it myself. Because it's quicker. And once they're under, I never let them up again."

I put my arm around her. No wonder she was so interested in Muriel Brackenbury's horrid death. If someone else had known the horrors of all those thrashings and struggles, and beads of air glistening to the surface, maybe she wasn't so alone.

I slid off the wall. Taking her hands in mine, I tugged at her gently.

"Come along, Tulip. Time to go home."

Then, one day, I heard the office staff discussing her.

"What *has* that child done with her hair?"

"Which?"

"Tulip Pierce."

I rooted deeper in the chest of lost property, hiding my face.

"Oh, *Tulip*."

They stared out of the window in silence for a while. Then one of them said,

"She is a strange one, that's for sure."

Her colleague sniffed.

"I can't be doing with her. Bold and sassy if you speak to her. But the minute she wants something from you, she turns into Miss Cute & Mincing."

"Have you seen her fingernails? They're bitten raw."

"I can't *think* what she's done to her hair. It looks as if someone's been at it with the garden shears."

The phone began ringing, and the nearest one turned from the window.

"My sister knows the mother," she remarked. "Just through her dealings with the farm." She reached out to press the flashing red button. "She says she always gets the feeling that one day she might start screaming and never stop."

I wondered who she meant. Tulip's mother? Or Tulip? And was this what the painting was about? Was this why Mrs Minniver, and everyone else, treated Tulip as if she were as dangerous as one of her own dustbin blazes?

Poke a fire, and it flares more fiercely. Everyone knows that.

The only safe thing is to stay away.

I think I almost came to the decision then. And maybe a dozen other times when I stepped out in early morning air, and knew I couldn't face her. On those days, I'd skip school myself, and spend the hours hiding in the Palace's abandoned laundry, where my footfalls raised puffs of dust, and I had to sit uncomfortably amid tubs and basins, in the shadow of a giant old mangle, watching a frill of light creep under the door.

At four o'clock, I'd make my way, out of sight, around the Palace to the bus stop. After a day in oily gloom, the great bars of sunlight sweeping so cleanly over the fields made me feel tearful and giddy.

I'd make sure Tulip was nowhere in sight.

Then I'd walk home, as usual.

Nine

TULIP WORE BLACK until it was taken from her.

"The colour for sweaters in this school is *blue*."

"But I'm wearing black for Muriel."

"Muriel?"

"Muriel Brackenbury."

You could tell that the teachers were disgusted. "Self-indulgence stretched into morbidity," said Mrs Powell. Mr Hapsley gave her a detention each time he saw her. And as soon as Miss Fowler was told, she stormed down the stairs from her office.

"Take off that pullover. It's confiscated."

"But I don't have another one with me."

"That's your problem, Tulip. Maybe tomorrow you'll wear proper uniform."

I found her waiting at the bus stop, shivering.

"Why didn't you go straight home?"

"I can't. I daren't. She said she'd be phoning my father."

So that's how I came to go on my last *Wild Night*. This time, it was a shed a mile out of town. I don't know where she'd got the paraffin. Maybe she'd sneaked it from home. I can't believe the people who owned that chicken farm were stupid enough to leave three whisky bottles filled with paraffin in a ditch on their own land.

"Tulip –"

"Ssh! If you can't help, at least don't spoil things by fussing."

"Are you quite sure it's empty?"

"You *know* it's empty. We've walked through it twice. Now pass me the last bottle."

The shed went up like nothing I've ever seen. Huge flames licked the sky, and smoke billowed up like a giant black genie freed from a bottle after thousands of years. The fire roared and crackled. Rafters collapsed like straws. And the dancing sparks spat and hissed as, one by one, the empty racks seethed and frizzled.

But this time it was Tulip tugging at my arm.

"Natalie! Natalie!"

I shook her off. The only thing I wanted was to

stand and watch this great orange dragon leap higher and higher.

"Natalie! Quick, or we'll get caught! The police always suspect everyone standing and watching!"

But, though she pulled at me, I wouldn't budge. Why go to all the trouble to raise a fire, and then not stay and watch? All round that chicken farm were hedges and hawthorn trees and clumps of bushes. If she'd been here before to stuff her bottles of paraffin into the ditch, surely she could have found some place we could have hidden. Why take so many risks, then walk away from all the glorious, spell-binding magic you've created? Why miss the fizzing, crackling glory of something so plain and drab exploding into fireballs and shooting stars?

"Oh, please, Natalie! Please!"

She tugged so hard at me, I had to go. But as I stumbled after her, still looking back, I knew I was bewitched. *The Tulip Touch* had really got me this time. I knew I'd dream of fires for ever, and wake in the middle of my dull, dark nights to see the flames she might have lit in me still shooting up to scorch the sky. I'd see whole streets, entire cities, burning. I'd switch on my bedside light and, for a while, the old familiar pictures on the walls and clothes on the chair might blot out the smouldering visions. But I'd be sure Tulip was lying waiting in some bleak bedroom. And I'd know the minute my room was dark again, she'd pick up where she left off, and send more of her own imaginings into my boring dreams, to set them ablaze with her own growing frenzies.

"Natalie? Natalie! Are you all right?"

I heard the whine of a siren. Was it in my head, or coming from across the field?

"Down here. Quick!"

She pushed my head below the level of the ditch, and stayed close behind me as we crept along.

"See that gap? That one!"

I crawled through the tiny hole in the hedge. She followed, and we lay on our backs, panting. I still felt dizzy and strange. And then, suddenly, out of the whirl of confusion came the first inklings of other, darker, more destructive visions.

And slowly, slowly, I came to my full senses at last.

Is it like this for everyone? Is it unusual to have your life bowling along steadily in one direction, and then, in a flash, change utterly? Change *everything*. For those were the moments when our friendship died. It's as easy as that to pin down. Oh, I let her rattle on, lifting her head to look at the fire engines, working out which way we ought to go back to the bus stop if we weren't to be noticed, talking excitedly about how fast that old wood flared up and burned. But all the time I was thinking, people *hide* in sheds. I'd spent whole days in the abandoned laundry. If someone I didn't know had walked through, I would have held my breath in the shadow of the huge, rusting mangle. And in the tension of the moment, even someone with hearing as good as mine might not have noticed the soft suspicious splatter of liquid on old trampled straw.

And what about Julius? He had a dozen dens. So did his friends. They hid for hours in outhouses so frail and rotten that, under the ivy that held them together, they would flare up in a moment.

Was Tulip *mad* as well as bad?

I clambered to my feet, and held out my hand as usual to pull her up.

"Come on, Tulip. Time to go home."

On the bus, she was her old, cocky self, flirting with the driver and slyly tipping people's shopping bags over with her feet.

Halfway back, she got restless.

"Want to play *All the Grey People*?"

"Sure," I said. And I did a good job of pretending

all the way. But when you've just won the hardest game of all, the others lose their colour. And so my heart wasn't in it, and it fell flat.

From the bus stop, we walked together to the bridge.

"Well," I said cheerfully. "See you tomorrow."

"Why don't I come as far as the Palace?"

I gave her a long look. She really hadn't realised I was out of it. She didn't know that she could never recast the spell.

"If you like," I said.

We strolled arm in arm up the drive. I felt quite calm. I wasn't worried in the least. And that, in itself, felt strange. It seemed that, from the day we'd met, I'd been in thrall to Tulip. Everything I'd said, everything I'd done, had her in mind. Like a tongue to a wobbly tooth, my every thought had come straight back to her. I had become a shadow to my parents. I'd floated out of reach of Julius. I had no friends. I hadn't been there for anyone, except for Tulip.

And it was over. All over.

I let her walk with me as far as the last bend in the drive. Then, as the Palace came in view, I broke away, and dropping my school bag, I ran as fast as I could across the rose garden, under the archway, and down the narrow twisty path snaked over with tree roots.

I heard her calling. "Natalie! *Natalie!*" But I didn't answer. I just ran. *Stay away from fire.* And when I'd reached the middle of the thicket, I came off the path and dived into the bracken.

I crawled and crawled. While she was thrashing between the trees, I'd make a little progress. Then when she was perfectly still, cunningly waiting, I didn't move at all.

"Natalie! *Natalie!*"

She was beating so fiercely at the undergrowth with a stick that I got a little further under the cover of her noise. And then even further, till I had reached our old mud slide. And down I went, down, down, sideways like a rolling log, faster and faster, until I came to rest in the very deepest bracken.

And there I lay, grinning up at the fronds that had closed over my head. She'd never find me now. I was safe in the green dark of jungle, of deep, deep, sunless pools. I lay on my back and listened as she called.

"Natalie! *Natalie!* Come out, stupid! It's raining!"

The first few drops pattered through the whispering fronds. The dripping turned into trickles, but I didn't move. Let her call. Let her search for me.

Let her give up and go home.

A soft bead of rain ran over my forehead and in my ear, and I recalled Miss Golightly, years before, explaining a picture in Assembly.

"He's pouring the water over the baby's head to put her on the side of light."

Tulip crashed nearer, but my heart stayed steady.

"Go away," I willed her silently, playing *The Tulip Touch* backwards for the very first time. "Turn around. Go away. I don't want you anywhere near me."

Not fire. *Light.*

She called a few more times, ever more hopelessly. And then she left.

PART
Three

One

IT WAS LIKE coming out of hospital. You don't get straight back into being yourself. It takes a little time. And just as someone with a broken foot gingerly tests it each morning to see how much pressure it can take, I stretched things a little further every day.

I had to be careful with Tulip. She was on her guard.

"What happened on Friday? Why did you run off like that?"

"Oh, I'm sorry. I suddenly felt so queasy. I knew I couldn't make it back to the Palace, so I ran off between the trees."

"Didn't you hear me calling?"

"I was *sick*."

The next day, she wanted to come home with me.

"We've got workmen," I told her. "And Dad says he doesn't want any extra visitors."

"What about the weekend?"

"There's a special wedding party."

"We could stay out of sight."

"No, Tulip."

She gave me a suspicious look. I knew how odd it must have sounded to her. She'd never heard me saying no before.

"You're hiding something, Natalie."

"No, I'm not."

"Well, something's going on. I used to be able to come, even when there were special parties and weddings."

I let the same look of dumb insolence spread over my face as I'd seen so often on hers.

"Well, that was last year, Tulip."

At this reminder of the game we used to play, she turned on her heel and walked off. I went back to my classroom, grinning. And it was only then I realised that, in this small daily probing of sides of myself left too long untested, I'd come across a few things I'd totally forgotten. The feeling of power. The sense of being in control.

Mr Scott Henderson was the first one to notice she was never around.

"Where's your friend Tulip these days? Have you two had a little spat?"

I looked unconcerned and lied glibly (both skills I'd learned from her).

"Not really. She's got other friends."

And soon she had. First she took up with Marcie once again, though that lasted only till the craze on playing cards began in break time. Then Marcie got fed up with Tulip's habit of going on about the rules through every hand, and telling everyone what they'd done wrong, and gloating over winning.

"It's just a game," she said. "It doesn't *matter*. Why do you care so much?"

Tulip's eyes flashed, and she stormed off. And after that she was alone again, till someone called Heather came down from Scotland and started at Talbot Harries. Like me, all those years ago, she didn't know any better than to offer her friendship to the first person she saw standing alone. And for the next few days I had to watch Tulip grin at me contemptuously, and turn her back, and giggle in corners with Heather.

But that didn't last, either. Heather soon took against Tulip's mean habit of eating the sweets she always had in her pocket without offering them to anyone round her. And Tulip's 'joke' of tipping the contents of Heather's lunchbox into the bin, and filling it with dirt and stones, fell very flat. So Heather soon made other friends. In any case, watching the two of them walk round together, arm in arm, hadn't made me unhappy. All I could see was how foolish I must have looked when it was me. All I could feel was sheer relief.

That was the strangest thing about those weeks: the feelings that I had. Like coming out of a grey, endless dream, I felt the world lift around me. For far too long, I'd stayed in Tulip's shadow. Each day now, I felt a bit stronger and things went better. At school, because I wasn't looking out for her on every staircase and through every window, my work was more careful and my marks improved. At the Palace, I walked more briskly in and out of rooms, no longer endlessly hovering by windows and doorways to see if Tulip was coming. Without half my brain engaged in waiting for her, I became a whole person again. At night I still dreamed of fires, and woke in frights. But in the day, so different did I feel, so little did I want to be the Natalie I was before, that I'd have changed my name if they'd have let me. And on the morning I found myself sitting peacefully on the ledge of the verandah, watching the peacocks instead of – one of the games she'd taught me – stalking them till they panicked, I realised for the first time in years that I was happy.

Happy.

And that's why, when Julius ran round the corner to tell me Tulip was waiting in the rose garden, I didn't want to know.

"Go back," I said, "and tell her you can't find me."

"Why?"

"Because I don't want to see her."

"But what about Tulip? If you're not with her, the gardener will tell her to go home."

I slid off the ledge and moved towards the door.

"Just tell her I can't come. Say that I'm busy helping Dad."

He looked baffled. But then he shrugged, and ran back the way he'd come. I felt a little bit guilty, but not much. Staying away from Tulip was getting easier each day.

And I avoided her at school as well. Skills learned in *Guest-stalk* came in useful now.

"Coming, or going, Natalie?"

I'd step aside to let the teacher pass. I didn't know yet, did I? If she was outside, I was staying in. If there was no sign of her, then I might slip out between the wide glass swing doors.

I'd have my bag packed by the end of school. I'd hare up Forest Street, though it was further, to catch the bus one stop ahead. I'd keep my head down as it roared past the gates, in case she was standing there waiting, or trailing her bag towards our usual stop in the vain hope I'd catch her up and keep her company. It wasn't my fault that she was alone. Nobody forced her to shove people so hard they fell, and splatter ink on their clothes, and call out "Cheap Scottish Heather!" all the time at someone who'd tried to be friendly.

Each time she came to the Palace, Julius told me off.

"You can't just keep saying you're busy."

"Yes, I can."

"You can't. It's mean. Tulip's supposed to be your friend."

"Just tell her I've gone to Urlingham with Mum. That's not so difficult, is it?"

"It's not that it's difficult," said Julius. "It's just that I feel sorry for her."

"Well, don't!" I snapped. "It's just a trap!"

He stared at me as if I'd bitten him.

"What do you mean?"

"Nothing," I said, getting a grip again. "I didn't mean it."

But I did. I was *sick* of feeling sorry for Tulip. I felt she'd caught me young, and sucked me in, and even made me bury my own feelings so deep, I practically didn't have them. She'd kept me down with her contempt and scorn. But things were different now. It was my turn to feel contempt. And I think I must have realised that part of my growing strength came from despising her, because I didn't stop at my new disapproval of her mad habits and her crooked ways. I took it a step further. Now, when we met in the corridors, I'd smile, and say hello, and mutter something about meeting at break. But at the same time, I'd be taking care to glance at the great lumpy hems on her second-hand school skirt, with all the ugly stitching showing through, or at the ragged hair she cut herself, so I could will myself to think:

"You're nothing, Tulip. *Nothing.*"

Oh, it was horrible. It was to save my life, but I could *weep*.

Two

SHE NEVER ASKED me what was wrong again. Sometimes I found my locker filled with litter, or my name on the "Commendation List" scratched out so hard it gouged the paintwork on the corridor wall. But I kept quiet about it to the teachers, and never said a word at home.

Still, even my parents must have noticed she never came. So I was really surprised when, halfway through December, Dad lifted his head from the Christmas seating plan to say to me,

"I take it Tulip's coming, as usual?"

I couldn't work it out at all.

"I'm not inviting her," I said.

He and Mum exchanged glances. Mum fiddled with the gold chain round her neck.

"But you know how much Tulip loves Christmas."

"I love Christmas as well," I said stubbornly. "And I don't feel like inviting her this year."

They looked uneasy. I got the feeling Dad was on the verge of telling me something, but, at a look from Mum, he changed his mind. Instead, he just said mildly,

"But she doesn't have much of a life, does she? So it might be nice."

Inside, I was seething. So that was it! I'd fought so hard to get free, yet here were both of them quite ready to throw me back, just to ease their own guilty consciences. They knew as well as I did she hadn't been in the Palace for weeks. But how could they feel as Christmassy as usual, if Tulip wasn't there, to make them feel even more giving and generous, with Dad feeding her titbits, and Mum whispering to the guests.

"Oh, yes. She has a pretty thin time of it at home. So we do try to give her at least one really special day."

Well, they couldn't have it both ways.

"Let Julius invite her," I said slyly. "She's really more his friend now."

"*Julius?*"

Mum was so startled, she almost snapped the necklace.

"Yes," I said. "They spend quite a bit of time together now. They're thick as thieves."

"Julius? And *Tulip*?"

Dad put his hand on Mum's to calm her down.

"I've never noticed," he said suspiciously.

"You're always very busy."

He let it drop. But Mum soon slid away to have a quiet word with Julius. I don't know what he said. But why should he have hidden the fact that, if he noticed Tulip on his way home from school, or saw her hanging round the edge of the cornfield, he always ran across to say hello? After all, he felt *sorry* for Tulip.

Didn't they all?

So my mean little plan to protect myself worked like a charm. Mum might not bother all that much about me, but when it came to looking after precious Julius, no one else stood a chance. The very thought of having Tulip for Christmas slipped out of everybody's mind, and no one said another word.

Except Mr Scott Henderson. At the piano on Christmas Eve, he poked me gently in the ribs.

"Are you missing her?"

"No," I said sourly, not even bothering to pretend I didn't know who he meant.

"I do," he said. "I've always had a soft spot for your little friend."

"She's not so little," I said. And then I thought of something cleverer. I put on a more pleasant face and turned to beam up at him.

"I could explain to you how to get to her house. Then, since you're so fond of her, you could go and visit."

That shut him up. He made great play of flicking through his carol sheet. Then, when the singing started, he kept his head bent to the words as if he didn't know them, and never caught my eye again.

I sang out, missing Tulip horribly, and hating them all. Why should they assume she was my job, always *my* job? They all knew where she was. They knew that she'd be sitting in her drab everyday clothes, listening to her mother hum and her father nag as she fingered some horrid cheap present scrimped from what was left of the housekeeping after Mr Pierce finished buying his booze. They all stood round the piano, so smug, so stuffed with food and so dolled up. What was so wrong with one of *them* filling a hamper and taking it over? Or even bringing her back with them? "Come on, Tulip. We know you're not best friends with Natalie any more. But *we* still care about you. Come with us."

But, no. That was *my* job. Look after Tulip (but don't be her hold-your-coat merchant). Be nice to her (but mind you don't get sucked in too far). Go play with the witch (but don't let her cast any spells on you).

Oh, dream on.

Three

DID SHE SIT there expecting us till the very last minute? ("Jump in, Tulip! Christmas is Christmas, after all.") Because, after that, there was no more pretending. When we met on the school stairs, she flashed me such a look of hate, and I stared past her coldly.

And with no friends, she went from bad to worse. I heard the whispers almost every day. "Did you know about Tulip? Guess what she's done now!" She hardly came in to school. And when she did, she had an air of smouldering anger around her. The boys picked up on it straight away, calling her 'Crazy Tulip' until the strange frozen mask on her face cracked, and she turned wild, and spun into frenzies of violence that had the phones ringing and the male staff running.

In February, she was banned from Harry's Supermarket. A few weeks after that, the police came in to school on her account. No one was sure exactly what it was about, but I realised I'd not known how much trouble she'd been in till I heard some of the guesses.

"It'll be because of those windows."

"Don't be soft. The police don't come round for smashed windows. Maybe she had the nerve to go back to Wilkins Hardware."

"To nick the batteries she forgot?"

They all laughed. I turned away, embarrassed, because even after all these months of steering clear of her, some of them still thought of me as Tulip's friend. And so did most of the teachers. Because it was to the Palace that the police were sent that very same night, pulling their caps off as they walked through the door, but ignoring the curious glances from the guests on the sofas.

Mum hurriedly ushered them away from Reception, and through the door into the office.

"You stay here, Natalie," she said. "Watch the desk for me, will you?"

The woman officer stood back to let me pass. But the man said,

"I think we might sort things out quicker if the young lady comes in as well."

"Really?" Mum was astonished. But she didn't argue. Instead, she called George in from the bar, and asked him to find someone to cover Reception.

"Now," she said, closing the door behind us all. "What's all this about? How can I help you?"

But they weren't to be hurried.

"Maria Benson," said the woman, offering her hand to Mum.

"Stallworthy," said the other, and smiled, though he made no effort to shake hands.

They glanced at the chairs till Mum said, "Please do sit down." And then they seated themselves, and looked at me. But I'd learned the blank face from Tulip. I didn't flinch.

"It's about some little visits," said the woman officer.

My heart began to thump. How long can your old life follow you? We couldn't have played *Little Visits* for nearly a year.

Mum was mystified. "Little visits?" She turned to me. "What little visits?"

I was so lucky. Before I could put my foot in it, Officer Benson broke in again, to try and explain.

"You see, we're having a little problem with Tulip Pierce."

"Oh, Tulip!" Mum's relief was evident. "Tulip! I might have known!"

"And we were wondering if Natalie here could help us understand."

I watched them warily, but it was Mum who asked.

"Understand what?"

"Why on earth she might be doing what she's doing."

Mum looked from one to the other.

"And what's that?"

The policeman picked at his cap. He seemed embarrassed suddenly, and tired.

"We've had a complaint. It seems Tulip has made three little visits to the family of that poor girl who drowned a while back. She keeps coming up to Mrs Brackenbury's door, and knocking, and asking her –"

He stopped, and seemed, for a moment, to be inspecting the plasterwork on the ceiling.

"Asking her –?" Mum prompted.

He took a deep breath.

"Asking if Muriel would like to come for a walk."

I saw Mum wasn't understanding yet. So did the officer. He tried again.

"Muriel Brackenbury," he explained. "The girl who drowned."

Mum's face went ugly with disgust.

"Tulip is *visiting* them? And asking after their dead child?"

"Standing there on the doorstep."

"Grinning all over her face."

"But that's disgusting! That's horrible! That is the worst, the sickest –"

She turned her anger and revulsion on me.

"Do you *hear* this? I hope I never again hear of you spending time with Tulip Pierce! Do you understand what these officers are *saying*?"

Officer Stallworthy broke in.

"That's why we're here, Mrs Barnes. Because –" He hesitated, perhaps fearing to focus Mum's wrath onto any particular gossips. "Because, when we asked around, we heard that Natalie may know Tulip well enough to help us understand exactly what it is we're dealing with here."

Mum's eyes were flashing.

"You want to know if Tulip's mad, or bad?"

His tired and embarrassed look came back again.

"That's not how we'd put it, of course. But if your daughter —" He turned to me. "Natalie, can you help us out? Can you tell us what's going on here?"

Oh, I did an excellent job. I looked so puzzled and anxious. I got more and more distressed. I shook my head, and started sentences I couldn't finish. And they must have thought I was being as open and honest as I could. You could see it on their faces. 'This girl is doing her level best to be some help.'

But all I let them know, through my pathetic stammered confidences, was that I'd stopped being friends with Tulip months ago, even before she took up with Marcie, and, afterwards, with Heather. Everyone could tell them that, I said. They could check it. But I told them nothing that they needed to know. I hadn't spent all that time building a wall between the old Natalie and the new to take it down now, for these two. So I never even tried to explain what was quite clear to me. Perfectly obvious.

If I'd been inventing games for two my whole life, and suddenly my old partner refused to play, what would there be to do but think up a whole load of new games, just for one?

And what a game! Here was I thinking our *Little Visits* had been so cool, so risky. And what was Tulip doing? Walking up to the mother of a dead girl and asking if her daughter could come out for a walk! Not just once, but three times in a row!

I was awestruck. She'd really left me standing, hadn't she? Here was I, playing Little Goody Two Shoes with Mum and Dad, and passing tests at school, and even spending hours with Julius. And here was she . . .

And once again I saw the old bewitching vision of how things could have been. The constant beat of excitement. Her hand in mine. And flickering, rising colours. Colours to light the sky, and warm my grey, grey soul, and fill my dreams for ever.

But standing there grinning, they'd said. Grinning all over her face.

At Muriel Brackenbury's *mother*.

Other people's feelings aren't dice, or counters.

"*Three times!*"

Officer Stallworthy took my belated disgust for astonishment, because he said a bit defensively:

"Well naturally, the first time, the Brackenburys thought it must be some horrible mistake."

"As anyone would," said Mum tartly.

"As anyone would," he repeated. "It was only the second time that they rang us." He paused. "And we made the same mistake. We just assumed that someone had got the wrong end of the stick. Upsetting, of course. But totally innocent."

Again, he stared at the ceiling.

"But then, this evening —"

This evening! Incredible! Less than three hours ago I'd spotted her from the bus as it swept past school. She'd looked the same as usual. But here were these two police officers saying she'd strolled up the path to a house (where, for all she knew, half of the county's squad cars were lying in wait for her after her first two visits) and treated another human being as if she were just part of some *game*.

"She's mad," said Mum. "There has to be something wrong with her. She's insane."

Officer Stallworthy decided the visit was over. He took a card from his breast pocket, and after hesitating between Mum and me, put it in my hand.

"Any time," he said gently. "Anything you can think of that might help. Anything at all."

I nodded.

They moved towards the door. Mum signalled me to stay behind, but still I distinctly heard her say,

"Honestly, I don't know what Natalie ever saw in Tulip Pierce."

Perhaps it was her dismissive tone that irritated Officer Stallworthy. Maybe, if you're in the police, you get a little tired of people in plushy surroundings telling you how they're above all the squalid little messes you spend your whole life sorting out.

Anyhow, he said rather coldly:

"Perhaps, Mrs Barnes, it's time to start wondering just what it was that Tulip saw in Natalie."

Mum just ignored the jibe. But to remind him who was supposed to be the villain here, she asked,

"And what is likely to happen to Tulip now?"

"Oh, we'll speak to her. She won't go bothering them again."

The wall I'd built so carefully broke. Not even caring that Mum would realise I'd been eavesdropping, I rushed through the door and caught him by the sleeve.

"Promise me you won't tell her father! Promise me!"

Mum looked first shocked, then disapproving.

"They'll have to speak to Tulip's parents, Natalie."

"No! Please!" I begged. "They mustn't! If they tell Mr Pierce, he'll *kill* her. I *know* he will!"

Officer Stallworthy said kindly,

"Don't you worry. We'll take it very gently. I think we all know about Mr Pierce's temper."

"No!" I cried, dragging at him, near hysterical, half dead with fright for Tulip. "You don't understand. If you tell him what she's been doing, he'll half murder her. He'll just be glad to have the chance. He'll sound reasonable enough while you're there. But the minute you're gone –"

The words came searing back from games we'd played together, things she'd said.

"The minute you're gone, he'll thrash her like a red-headed stepchild! He'll whip her till her freckles sing!"

They stared at me, appalled. Even my mother was silent.

The officers eyed one another, said nothing, and were gone.

Four

NEWS TRAVELS FAST in a hotel. Mum didn't say a word to me, but she must have spoken to someone, because the very next evening I walked through the lounge to hear the argument raging around me.

"Wickedness!" Miss Ferguson was saying. "Pure *wickedness!*"

"Nonsense," said Mrs Pettifer. "The child is obviously deeply disturbed."

Instead of moving on through the double doors, I drifted to a halt out of sight behind one of the pillars, to listen. As usual, Mr Enderby tried to keep the peace.

"It might have been a misunderstanding. That's always possible."

"Oh, really!" snapped Miss Ferguson. "It's perfectly obvious that that Pierce girl is malevolent by nature."

Julius looked up from the spelling book he was pretending to study.

"Are you talking about Tulip?"

Mrs Pettifer couldn't order Miss Ferguson to be quiet. Instead, she sent Julius out of the lounge.

"Off you go, dear. I'm sure you can't be doing your homework properly here."

Julius trailed away, probably glad of the excuse to give up on his spellings. I expect Mrs Pettifer glanced round to check I wasn't listening, either. But I was well hidden. So by the time that Mum came over to have a few words with them before dinner, the three had started up again.

"I was just telling Mrs Pettifer," said Miss Ferguson, "that part of the problem for children today is that they hear far too many people like herself telling them they understand all their problems, and not enough like me stating quite openly that some of their behaviour is downright evil."

Old Mr Hearns had kept dead quiet up till then. He'd probably been hoping that this discussion would die away, and he'd be asked to play the piano, as usual. But now he got irritated, and spoke up.

"Oh, I see! They're bad seeds, are they? Spawn of the devil?"

She missed his sarcasm entirely.

"That's right!" she said. "And when I was a girl, these things were made perfectly clear to us. We even had to learn a little poem. 'Satan is glad when I am bad.'"

"Oh, I know that one!"

This was Mr Scott Henderson, who winked at me as he strolled in behind George, who was carrying a tray of drinks from the bar. Rumbled, I stepped out from behind the pillar. But no one noticed me. They were still busy looking at Mr Scott Henderson, who had clasped his hands together, and started declaiming:

> "'Satan is glad
> When I am bad
> And hopes that I
> With him shall lie
> In fire and chains
> And awful pains.'"

"Hardly a *poem*," Mr Hearns muttered critically. But Mum took the chance to stop the argument in its tracks by starting a small storm of clapping. Mr Scott Henderson took a bow. And after a 'please break it up' eye-signal from Mum, George made a point of giving everyone the wrong drinks. In the confusion that followed, Mum leaned over the arm of Mr Hearns's chair, and said softly:

"I think a tune would be nice now, don't you?"

Gratefully, he rose and launched into what I've often heard Mum call 'that awful stale medley of his'. Mum kept the smile fixed on her face, and nodded to the music. And she was still determinedly humming 'Bye-Bye Blackbird' when the grandfather clock took to striking its arthritic half hour, and all of them finally prised themselves out of their armchairs and off their sofas, and wandered across the lobby, into the dining room.

Mum's bright look crumpled like a dead balloon. Leaning her head against the chair back, she closed her eyes. I thought she might call me over to talk about the visit from the police, and what I'd said about Tulip's father. But, within seconds, the telephone outside was ringing again. She waited and waited. And when it was obvious that none of the staff was close enough to take it, she sighed and levered herself to her feet.

A few moments later, she was gone.

Five

S HE WOULDN'T LET the guests get into fights. But upstairs she and Dad went at it hammer and tongs.

"Miss Ferguson's quite right. Tulip is downright *evil*."

"I can't believe I'm hearing you right, Emma. You know those old biddies down there are light years from knowing the first thing about children. No one is born evil. No one. And especially not Tulip."

Mum turned away to tip stale flower water in the sink, and run in fresh.

"I don't know how else you'd explain something so horrible."

"Oh, don't be so silly. You know as well as I do that Tulip's had such a rotten start in life that it's hardly a surprise she's insensitive to other people's feelings."

"There's a bit more to this than being insensitive!" snapped Mum, slamming the vase back on the table.

He reached out to steady it.

"You know what I mean. To really know right from wrong you need a certain emotional sympathy. And you only learn that from being treated properly yourself."

"Tulip's not stupid. Tulip knows the rules."

"Why should she think rules matter? Her father's are vindictive and wilful, and sometimes it must seem to her that, whatever she does, she gets punished. So why should she bother about rules?"

I had to keep myself from turning round. I'd no idea, before this argument, that they knew so much about Tulip.

"Why should she bother? Because she's bright enough to see that if enough people like her go round doing exactly what they want, *everyone's* miserable."

"If you've been brought up as if your feelings don't matter, you probably assume other people's don't matter much either."

In the corner, Julius's computer game chattered to its climax. Mum's voice rose above it.

"Don't kid yourself, Martin! Tulip knows perfectly well how much other people's feelings matter. And that's exactly why she does these things. That's the amusement she gets from them. Why else would she do it?"

Dad couldn't think of an answer. He just shrugged. And then, reluctant to give up his defence of Tulip, he said:

"Well, you only have to pick up a paper to read about kids a lot younger doing worse."

To prove his point, he read Mum a paragraph from the *Chronicle* lying on the table about the murder of a boy in Elvenwater where the police were quite sure that the killer was no older than the victim. I don't remember the details. Something to do with footprints, and a squabble overheard by somebody pegging out washing, and too many people noticing two young people going down the path, only one coming back. I do remember the police were certain. The one they were looking for was even younger than me.

Mum listened, but she wouldn't budge.

"Children with violent tempers, I can understand," she said. "Even children with too few brains to realise how dangerous a game is getting. But Tulip's visits to the Brackenburys are out of another box entirely. They're not just bad. They're different. And that's what evil is. Something *different*."

"There's no such thing as evil. You know that."

And round and round they went, round and round, while I leaned over Julius's shoulder, and pretended to be absorbed in his fast-rising score. Mum had barely begun on the vase on the side table before Dad was arguing with her again.

"Look, Emma. Even professionals come across the odd child they just can't stand. The child they can't help thinking is deeply, deeply mean inside. And then what usually happens is that they meet the parents. And they begin to think, 'Poor little brute. No wonder the child's such a horror.'"

"Oh, right!" scoffed Mum. "Then I've got a brilliant idea. Why don't you take Mr and Mrs Pierce round to meet Mrs Brackenbury? Then she can start feeling sorry for Tulip."

That shut Dad up.

"*See?*" Mum said, and walked past him into the bathroom, carrying the misting spray. She made a point of letting the door close behind her.

The buzzer from downstairs rang twice.

Dad pushed himself up from the table. Seeing me

watching, he pushed the newspaper over the table towards me, and said darkly:

"Good thing that Tulip has an alibi!"

It was a joke. But what he didn't know was that, after the paper came, I'd spent a good half hour kneeling on the chest in the passage, scouring the map for Elvenwater, checking the scale, and doing the calculation over and over, till I was absolutely sure.

Six

AND IT WASN'T the first time, either. Ever since the blaze at the chicken farm, I'd scoured the evening paper every night. As I came in from school, Dad would lift his head from the computer, or turn from the rack of numbered room keys.

"Be an angel, Natalie. Take round the papers."

I'd scoop the pile of *Chronicles* into my arms. And round I'd go. Slap, slap. One on every second sofa. Slap. Three on the menu table. Two in the bar. Two in the coffee room. All the rest in the lounge.

Except for the one I took up to my bedroom. I read the whole thing. Thefts. Beatings. Vandalism. I'd dutifully turn each page. **FIRE INJURES HOMELESS MAN**. The usual thing. They must print stories like it ten times a week. A garbled account from someone passing by of how he smelled the smoke and saw the flames. And, just above, a picture of a burnt-out shed. I'd try to tell myself a drunk tramp nearly died in a fire, and that was that. Just because Tulip lit fires, it didn't follow that she started this one.

But still she'd be my chief suspect. Sometimes I'd be so convinced that it was her, I'd have to stop and read the report again. Only then would I see the words 'Wednesday lunchtime' and remind myself that I'd seen her flouncing into detention at that time. 'The suspect was male,' I'd notice on second reading. 'The suspect is six feet tall.'

And who were they, anyway, these people who filled up the pages of the *Chronicle*, night after night? Were they all like Tulip, living life as one game after another? Tire of one, and move on to another even harder and more dangerous? They couldn't all have fathers as vile and bullying as Mr Pierce, and mothers too feeble to protect them. Surely there weren't that many horrid people in the world. And, if there were, I wasn't sure I wanted to go on buses any more, or walk down streets, for fear of bumping into them.

Dad found me in the passage once too often.

"Quite the little cartographer," he said as he passed.

"What?"

"Maps," he called over his shoulder. "Each time I

see you these days, you're kneeling on that chest, studying the map."

"I was just checking something."

Suddenly he stopped, and put the television he was carrying down on the floor.

"Room 302," he said. "Don't let me forget." Then he sat on the chest beside me and pushed my hair out of my eyes.

"Is something worrying you, Natalie? Is there anything wrong?"

Everyone has choices. I'd shied away from him time and again because, close to Tulip, I didn't need him. Tulip's touch was enough. But now she wasn't there, I realised I'd been hiding from both my parents. I'd used the fact that they were busy, and Mum was so wrapped up in Julius, to slip away from them and keep them off me. And it had worked. If you're a good girl, and dress neatly, and do your homework, no one will even notice you. You can leave a pretend person in your place to say 'Good morning', and pass the beans, and carry the dishes to the hatch. If they're not looking, then they'll never know.

Or you can raise a hand to save yourself. Make sure they see you.

"I was just looking at the map," I said. "To work

out if it could be Tulip who stabbed that old lady on Thursday in Bridleford."

He turned to stare.

"*What?*"

I kept my voice steady.

"But that lady was stabbed and robbed at three o'clock, the police say. And we didn't finish with the school photo till after two-thirty. And Bridleford's miles away." I showed him, to scale, with my fingers. "And Tulip has no bike. So I reckon Tulip has an alibi."

He was still staring.

"Is this what you've been doing each time I've seen you on this trunk?"

I nodded.

He shook his head in amazement.

"But why on earth would you think it was Tulip?"

"Well, tell me," I said. "Who are these people, if they're not people like her?"

"Listen," he said. "This is ridiculous. I know Tulip's turning into a bit of a bad lot, but –"

I interrupted him.

"You were around at lunch. You heard Mrs Pettifer telling everyone what the policeman told his wife."

Dad looked irritated.

"Gossip! Rubbishy gossip! These old biddies should keep their mouths shut."

But I knew he knew better.

"'It isn't a home,' he told her. 'That house is just a cold shell keeping the rain off three people. I was there half an hour,' he said. 'And the only real life in there was that great big dog barking.'"

Dad sighed.

"Oh, dear. Poor Tulip."

That wasn't going to wash. I turned on him accusingly.

"And you knew that. You've known it years and years. That's why you never let me go round there, even at the start. Even back then I heard you telling Mum it was –" I imitated his stern voice. "'No fit place for a child.'"

"Well, then," he said rather smugly. "I was right."

"But *Tulip* was a child, wasn't she? If you were so sure I shouldn't have been there, then Tulip shouldn't have been there, either."

"Natalie, people can't go round snatching children and giving them other homes just because their parents are awful."

"She shouldn't have been left," I said stubbornly.

He tried to take my hand.

"You really mustn't think that nobody tried. I know for a fact we weren't the only ones to make a few warning phone calls. And both schools were always well aware of Tulip's background. The Pierces have had social workers round there time and again."

So everybody was in it! Everyone knew!

"So what was the matter?" I asked sarcastically. "Wasn't it bad enough?"

He rose to his feet and looked down at me.

"No," he said evenly after a moment. "It wasn't bad enough. And I'm afraid that life's a bit like that, Natalie. It has to be a whole lot worse than bad to count as unbearable. And, till it gets to that point, people are on their own."

I was disgusted. Utterly disgusted.

"They've got to stick up for themselves, have they?" I said scornfully. "Manage on their own?"

He paused. Then,

"Why not?" His voice was still even. "You've heard Mrs Pettifer say it often enough. 'Every saint has a past. Every sinner has a future.' And you've even managed it yourself. Look at you. No more warnings on your report cards. No more lost hours after school. Better marks. Better habits. You've let down Tulip and you've saved yourself."

I wanted to scream at him. "Yes, but I'm not like you, am I? I've got no power to change things. You lot *have*."

But what would have been the point? He couldn't afford to believe me. None of them could. That way, they'd have to feel as guilty as me.

So I didn't say anything. I just nodded at the television he'd left on the floor.

"Don't forget," I said. "You're going to Room 302."

"Oh, right."

He took the hint then, and he walked away.

Seven

AND AFTER THAT, I put Tulip Pierce out of my mind, and got on with my own life. This time I did it properly. I spent my break-times in the library, gradually daring to take a seat nearer and nearer one of the small gangs of girls who sat together, till one day Glenys asked if she could borrow my protractor, and Anna told me that she liked my hair.

And from then on, I joined them in the lunch queue every day, and walked to the bus stop with Glenys. A week or so later, when she was chatting about the party she was planning at the weekend, she asked me, "Why don't you come too?"

And I was in at last.

I still saw Tulip in the corridors, on days she came.

And, like the rest of them, I took an interest in her foul-tempered brushes with the staff, and all her defiant rebellions.

"Did you hear what she called Mrs Minniver? Everyone's saying she'll be asked to leave."

"My dad heard that she'd been reported to the police for slashing the bus seats."

"It wasn't bus seats. It was theft."

Tulip stormed up the staircases, and in and out of rooms, snarling at everyone.

"Move out of the way, idiot!"

And most of them did. She made almost everyone nervous. I think they all thought that someone the staff could barely pretend to control was far too dangerous even to stand near. The trouble she got in, instead of curbing her, seemed to make her worse. She became more and more insolent, almost insanely cocksure. Indifferent to threats and warnings, even to punishment, she took her continual suspensions in her stride. We'd see her swaggering out between the gates at all hours of the day, and not be able to begin to guess whether she'd been sent home officially, or just decided it was time to go.

But, as her reputation grew, so did mine. In March, I passed all my exams so well I was commended. Miss

Fowler called in my parents and told them she was moving me into a different stream.

"It will be hard," she said. "But Natalie is doing so well, I'm sure she'll manage."

And I did. Easily. Somehow, the harder I worked, the more I enjoyed it. And when, at the end of the school year, I won three of the prizes and had to walk across the stage in front of everyone to take my books and shake Miss Fowler's hand, I realised Tulip and I had now reached equal distinction in our separate ways. Everyone knew me for an excellent pupil. And everyone knew her for a bad lot.

And then I bumped into her in the cloakroom.

"Move over, stupid!" she snapped at me, pushing past.

Perhaps she'd called me that once too often when we were younger. Or maybe, still carrying my brand-new prizes, I wasn't ready to be insulted any more.

Anyhow, stupid I was. Deliberately, quite deliberately, I let my eyes slide off her face, down her stained pullover to her puckered skirt.

And wrinkled my nose.

One look in her eyes, and I knew I'd gone far too far.

"Oh, so we're playing games again, are we?"

Hastily, I tried to backtrack.

"I don't know what you mean."

She just ignored me.

"We haven't played one for ages, have we, Natalie? What do you feel like? *Hogs in a Tunnel*? *Havoc*? *Road of Bones*? How about *Watch the Skies*? You always enjoyed that."

I'd never realised eyes could go so hard. Suddenly I felt sick with fright.

"Leave me alone, Tulip!"

She made her eyes go wide.

"That's not very nice, is it? After all, you were the one to start."

"I haven't started anything."

"Yes, you have. You just began with *Stinking Mackerel*. I saw you."

Nobody knows you like your old best friend. There was no point in saying anything. I just made for the door.

"That's agreed, is it?" she called after me. "Now it's my turn to choose."

I pretended I wasn't listening. Tugging the swing doors to make them close faster behind me, I hurried down the long corridor to get away. When, at the corner, I glanced back, she wasn't behind me. But that wasn't any comfort. After all, she had no need to follow me herself. Her menacing little words were doing that.

I rushed into the safety of my next class, and took my seat, my heart thumping. Nobody looked my way. Nobody noticed. But I sat there in terror. I knew Tulip. And, deep inside, not only did I know that she'd not rest till she'd won the very last game of all. I also knew exactly which of them she'd choose.

Eight

THE NEXT FEW days, I felt like that poor trembling rabbit in Tulip's clutch, waiting for something to happen. But one week turned into two, then three, and Tulip never even glanced my way. And then, at the end of the next week, the holidays started.

Time and again, that summer, I checked with Julius.

"You haven't seen Tulip hanging around anywhere, have you?"

He'd look up from whatever he was doing.

"Tulip? No. Why? Is she coming round?"

"I don't think so. But if you see her, will you let me know?"

I'd try not to sound worried, and maybe that was a mistake. Because once, when I asked him, I got a different answer.

"I thought I saw her a couple of days ago, by the old

garages. But when I called her, she just disappeared."

"Next time, tell me straight away, will you?"

"If you like."

I searched the garages, but found nothing. And, looking back, I'm not surprised. Tulip was cleverer than that. The days went by. Dad started paying me for little jobs, and Mum needed help in the office, so I was kept busy. Glenys came over once or twice, and I went to her house. And gradually I let myself believe that all Tulip had in mind that day was making me nervous. She knew exactly how faint-hearted I could be. What could be smarter than leaving me to worry, week after week, about something she'd long forgotten?

And so I let myself stop fretting. There was so much to do. When school term began again after the summer, I had a whole lot more work and netball practice twice a week. I got a part in the school play, and what with the flurry of extra rehearsals after half term, before I could believe it, Christmas was on its way again.

"Are you inviting Glenys?"

"No," I said. "She's off to her dad's house."

"How about Anna, then?"

"She says her mum would have a fit if she went to someone else for Christmas."

Dad shrugged.

"Makes sense. I wouldn't like it if you were away."

So I was there. There in my new green skirt through all the sherries and the canapés. There through Mr Hearns's Christmas medley on the piano. There through the charity raffle.

And there through the carols, as usual, with Julius bravely singing the first verse of *Once in Royal David's City* all alone, and Mrs Scott Henderson chiming in on every last verse with her ghastly descants, and Mr Hearns faltering even more than usual because he'd mislaid his glasses. The guests sang out, their faces winking from brightness to shadow as, through the french windows, the coloured lights along the terraces blinked on and off, on and off, over and over.

Oh, clever, clever Tulip! To pick the one evening everyone's in the same room, and all the kitchen staff who haven't managed to persuade Dad they're not needed are running round in circles, or peering into special soups, or diving into ovens to check on yet another difficult dish. Clever, clever Tulip, to pick the only night no one's around to see a small dark figure pouring petrol, and paraffin, and God knows what else, on all the sills and lintels, all the doors and benches, railings and signs, everything wooden round an old hotel.

And clever Tulip, to give herself a good head start. To choose the night when no one is going to notice, till it's far too late, that the sherry-flushed faces in the firelight are blinking pinker and brighter, pinker and brighter.

"Fire! Fire! Outside on the verandah! *Fire!*"

Alarms went off as the first flames broke through. The sprinkler system Dad put in the year we came spun into action at once. Everyone did the right thing. Nobody panicked. The guests, as Mum said afterwards, were "Marvellous! Marvellous!" They gathered on the lawns, and ticked each other off on lists as though they'd been in fires all their lives. No one sneaked back inside to fetch their jewellery. No one played daft heroics for the cat. And though Cedric had to be dragged away from the oven in which his *Boeufs en Croute* were crisping up nicely, all the kitchen staff switched off their grills and their gas jets in an orderly fashion, and left immediately through the nearest doors.

So by the time the first of Tulip's carefully primed explosions shattered the glass in the conservatory, everyone was safely out, watching the flames take hold. And if she hadn't thought to dig away the leaf mould of a hundred years to drag closed the giant iron gates at the bottom of the drive (and loop them round with so many chains and padlocks that the firemen believed her when she called out to them, "No! Not these gates! The other ones. Round there!"), then the first fire engine wouldn't have got bogged down in the muddy lane leading to their farm, and the second one would have broken in just that much quicker.

And so the Palace burned. Julius and I stood side by side to watch. His face flared in the fire's dancing light as one dark framed window after another burst into a fierce glow.

He turned to me, his cheeks burning as much with excitement as the reflection of the flames.

"Was it Tulip?"

My face was probably as flushed as his as I began the long, long lie.

"Now how on earth should I know?"

Cheerfully, he turned back to the blaze to watch the firemen send their huge coils of water snaking over the parapets. Like Tulip's stolen gold necklace hurled in the rubbish drum all that time ago, they slithered into the building's giant shell, and vanished instantly. I wondered, was she watching too? How did it feel, to see the only place she ever loved go up in flames? Inside, the dimpled copper bar top she used to stroke was buckling and melting. The glorious curving banisters she trailed her fingers up a million times were twisting to ugly shapes as they charred. Did she *care*? Was she hidden up somewhere in a tree behind us, just like one more roosting peacock, crying her eyes out? Or had she simply laughed, and run off home for yet another beating for being late?

Dad came up behind, and rested his hands on our shoulders. He couldn't say a word. He just stood there and watched. And so did Mum. We stood in silence as the Palace gradually gave up the fight, and out of the deafening hissing and spitting and crackling and roaring, the silent billows of smoke curled away in defeat over the huge dark spinney where Tulip had crept to hide her dangerous little toys week after week, till she was ready to play the very last, very worst, game of all.

Nine

SO NOW WE'RE off. Tomorrow we leave for Nettle Underwood. *The Starbuck Arms*. Dad's pretty cheerful about it. Sometimes you'd think that Tulip had done him a favour.

"These grand old buildings like the Palace have had their day," he keeps telling everyone. "Too many planning rules. Hotels that size can't stay afloat with just a few loyal regulars and passing tourists. These days you really have to be up-to-date. Health centres. Swimming pools. A proper dance floor. Lifts to every floor. They've got all those at the Starbuck."

Mum's come to terms with losing so many things. She had a weep about some photographs that were ruined (mostly because they were ones of Julius, I expect). And there were a couple of phone calls with the insurance people that left her shaking with rage. But yesterday she looked round the mess and clutter in the room where she's dumped all we have left, and said to me,

"Nothing worth dusting. Nothing worth bothering about. Come for a walk with me, Natalie. Let's go and have coffee together in the village."

And no one there minds much. Drinks at the hotel were always too expensive for most of the people round here. And the company's selling the site to someone who wants to build nice modern houses. So they don't mind, either. They're not blaming Dad. After all, he's never made a serious mistake before. And though an accidental fire should have been stopped at the outset, everyone's agreed that arson's another matter.

I worried terribly about Julius. But it turns out he doesn't care a hoot. He won't say anything in front of them, but to me he's admitted it. He enjoyed the fire. "Brilliant!" he calls it. He's become famous at school, describing it over and over. And though we're leaving now, he says he never wanted to move on to Talbot Harries anyway. He's glad he's going to another school.

And so am I. Everyone needs the chance to start again. Though I was doing pretty well, it seems. I know because on Friday, Miss Fowler called me in to show me the report she's sending on to Nettle

Underwood. 'After a period of confusion, Natalie Barnes has made a prodigious effort to find herself. She should go on to better and better things, and we all wish her well.' I told Glenys we were leaving, and promised her that I'd write every week. But, if I'm honest, I'll miss her less than the stone boy in the lily pond. She's never been a close friend.

Not like Tulip.

I don't think I'll be seeing her again. Her name comes up the whole time, of course, what with the gossip about the police enquiry, and the probation officer's report. Mum calls her "That witch Tulip!" and Dad says "Nonsense, Emma!" every time. But I can't help but think that being a real witch would have been better for her. At least that way she'd have a little power. Tulip's got nothing now. Yesterday, when we were packing, Julius asked me,

"If you could rub Tulip out of your past life, would you do it?"

And I had to shake my head. I can't regret the times we had together. Sometimes I worry I won't have times like that again, that there will be no lit nights, no incandescent days. But I know it's not true. There can be colour in a million ways. I know I'll find it on my own.

I have strange dreams about her. Sometimes the two of us are sitting cross-legged in one of the out-houses behind her farm, stirring a liquid we call 'flame-water', or crawling on our bellies through an orchard, trying to set fire to the flowers. But mostly, when I dream, Tulip and I are back in our first school, giggling and being silly, or lying on our backs behind the parapet, our bare arms touching, playing *Watch the Skies*.

I think about the day that Dad and I first saw her in that field of corn, and try to tell myself it was already too late. There's no particular moment when someone goes to the bad. Each horrible thing that happens makes a difference, and there had probably been too many of those already in Tulip's life.

But I can't convince myself. Yes, now I know that even back then, Tulip was going off to drown that poor kitten. But Dad was no older the day he pushed his grandfather's tortoise under the bush and left it there to die. You could say that Tulip was braver and kinder. And people aren't locked doors. You can get through to them if you want.

But no one did. No one reached out a hand to Tulip. Nobody tried to touch her. I hear them whispering and they sicken me. "Bus seats!" grumbles

Mrs Bodell. "Locker doors!" complain the teachers. "Chicken sheds!" say the farmers. "Greenhouses! Dustbins!" moan the neighbours. And Mum says, "A lovely old hotel!"

But what about Tulip?

I shall feel sorry for Tulip all my life.

And guilty, too.

Guilty.